Raffi Yaakobi

A Friendly Change

Raffi Yaakobi

A Friendly Change

Senior Editors & Producers: Contento
Illustrations: Yigal Vardi
Portrait: Mosha Yozefpolsey
Translator: Keren Druyak
Editor: Yosef Bloch
Cover and Book Design: Liliya Lev Ari

Copyright © 2015 by Raffi Yaakobi and Contento

All rights reserved. No part of this book may be translated, reproduced, stored in a retrieval system or transmitted, in any form or by any means, electronic, photocopying, recording or otherwise, without prior permission in writing from the author and publisher.

ISBN: 978-197-566-866-2

International sole distributor: Contento
22 Isserles Street, 6701457 Tel Aviv, Israel

www.ContentoNow.com
netanel@contento-publishing.com

Raffi Yaakobi

A Friendly Change

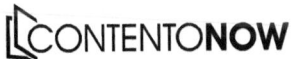

Table of Contents:

Friendship School: The Gist of the Method 7
Introduction: Everyone Can Change 35

Part 1 41

Chapter 1: Towards Change – The Friendly Change 43
Chapter 2: Your Brain as Your Friend 48
Chapter 3: Canonical Psychology and the Treadmill Culture 68
Chapter 4: Doing Things Differently: The Learning Culture 78
Chapter 5: Yes We Can 97
Chapter 6: Identity Changes – Navigating the Sea of Opportunities ... 110

Part 2 131

Chapter 7: Shaping and Changing our Daily Lives 133
Chapter 8: Changing Our Relationship Ability –
From a Single to a Spouse 153
Chapter 9: Changing the Relationship – Learning to Be Friends 174
Chapter 10: Change in Sex Life – From a Kitten to a Tiger 202
Chapter 11: Change with Children – Growing with the Child 211
Chapter 12: Change with Adolescents – Busting the Myth 234
Chapter 13: Never Stop Changing 250
Chapter 14: The First Meeting is the Most Important 264
Chapter 15: The Second Meeting 281
Chapter 16: The Next Meetings 287
Chapter 17: The Partner Gets Involved 296
Chapter 18: Some Parting Words 305
Glossary 309

Friendship School:
The Gist of the Method

I have been a psychologist for many years. I was educated and introduced into the profession as a clinical, psycho-dynamic psychologist. In my continuing efforts to assist my clients, I gradually became aware that the common therapy procedure which is based on diagnosing and then treating problems and symptoms usually turned into a hothouse of frustrating fixations and repetition. Unfortunately, as time passed, I came to the conclusion that, even if people **did** change during the treatment period, they did it despite the treatment and not as a result of it. In other words, those who started off with fierce, irresistible urges to grow and evolve, continued to develop, even if they continued to obey the principles of therapeutic culture, that is to bring up memories, discuss matters they were concerned with and describe their feelings and emotions in minute detail. However, those who started therapy with a certain developmental difficulty and started discussing their weaknesses and frustration with an attentive, sympathetic therapist, recycled their inhibitions. They tended to define themselves as people who have problems and came up with a variety of insights and reasons that explain and justify their numerous problems and therapy became the center of their world. Moreover, they used the same tools and the same landscape to diagnose their friends, their spouses and their children – this was a cultural blow.

Thus, most treatment methods serve the common characteristics in human nature, contribute to the fixation and diminution of people's worlds and sabotage the prospect of change. Some methods manage to create an illusion of change.

For the sake of those of you who resent my attacks on their beliefs, I must say that I do not make do with attacks, but I have created a much more efficient method which I must share with you. The method is about acquiring tools for realizing human potential, and tools that enable people to expose themselves to a diversified, ever-changing world, to find their way within it and even influence it.

It is possible that I was one of the first coaches in the world to have created a new, totally original method, which I called "Friendship School." The term 'school' offers learning, instead of treating, as a means of producing change, while 'friendship' is an art which one should learn as soon as possible. The art of friendship is the basis of success in relationships between spouses, parents and children, businesses, and even between countries. In other words, the method is a world view; it also contributes to a way of thinking which enables us to use our brain in the most effective way.

So far I have published five best sellers: : *"How to Learn Friendship," "The Friendly Psychologist," "Be Friends with your Children," "To Make a Couple"* and *"Friendly Change."* All of my books are about learning how to think.

The method has proved itself to be remarkably effective and in most cases has resulted in changes within short periods of time. It evolved from the rich and varied experiences acquired during many years of work. as well as accumulated documented successes.

Indeed, a person who has lived for many years in a non-scholastic culture finds it difficult, at first, to acquire the tools of friendly thinking, just as adults usually find it difficult to start learning a new language.

In the traditional therapeutic approach physicians tend to seek all sorts of symptoms that indicate problems and then make a diagnosis. They also seek to understand the reason for the formation of the problem and then treat it. According to the traditional approach, we must, first of all, define the problem, then understand its sources, and finally solve it – only then can we move on. But, there is always the danger of wasting tremendous effort or causing damage to a person who perceives himself as one who has problems and needs therapy. This diagnostic, analytic thinking is effective when examining electrical appliances or car engines. Identifying the problem and its sources provide the solution. On the other hand, people require a different type of thinking. They require creative and friendly thinking. In "Friendship School" we are aware of the fact that reality is extremely diversified and varied, so that more creative channels of solutions can be found within it. We bypass the symptom or the so-called problem and determinately move towards a friendly goal. A person who does that soon discovers that the new experience, which develops his ability, replaces the symptom. The things that were difficult become easy and the things that were frightening become enjoyable, and so forth.

My Alternative to Diagnosis

I suggest scanning the human scenery and the field of opportunities. First, we refer to the reservoir of abilities which every person has. That is, we will examine all of the things the person does: starting with work – and ending with hobbies and other daily activities. In addition, we will refer to the things that we have accomplished. In other words, we will refer to his reservoir of abilities.

Frequently, existing elements overshadow desirable and potential elements. So it is necessary to view the scope of opportunities the person is exposed to. Obviously, the world is made up from much more opportunities than we can possibly seize. Thus we will deal with fascinating questions such as: What is in the best interest of that person? Which elements are friendly and worthwhile as far as he is concerned? In order to answer these questions we should learn how to filter the opportunities and choose the ones that will enable him maximal expression of his abilities. It is not a choice between good and bad, but a choice between good and better.

The idea behind promoting abilities as an alternative to dealing with problems. It is a means of channeling our energy towards the goal through change. This is done in an efficient, economical manner which is based on recruiting all human strengths for learning and practical experiences and by not dwelling on problems.

Learning as a Means

Change is produced through learning. Learning means not sticking with the things we are used to doing and like to do, but to develop new abilities despite the challenges involved. A person who only does the things he likes and is used to tends to get stuck in the same place. Sometimes such a person moves sideways instead of forwards; i.e. starts developing an ability, and then neglects it, starts something new, neglects it too and so forth. Every now and then he feels tired of something he has, and desires something new. On the other hand, a person who is a diligent student shapes his own identity and produces desirable changes. It is not enough to learn how to drive; a person must also get used to driving a car. It is not enough to learn how to play a musical instrument; a person must be persistent in playing. It is not enough to lose weight; a person must keep in shape and maintain his/her body.

Symptoms

Psychology copied medical thinking, which focuses on symptoms of diseases as a means to cure patients. In the therapeutic culture people are defined in terms of pathology and illnesses: they are anxious, neurotic, dyslexic and so forth.

In "Friendship School" we do not focus on the symptoms but on the person's abilities. We define people according to their profession, their marital status and hobbies. In this method we refer to symptoms as side effects which are similar to new beginnings.

In other words, starting to learn a new ability sometimes involves difficulties and symptoms, but down the road, when the ability is established and joins the other components of identity – the symptoms vanish and are replaced with enjoyment and a sense of fulfillment.

Many people rush into diagnosing themselves according to their immediate, initial sensational response: "It is not for me" – and give up on the change. On the other hand, in the scholastic culture we bypass the symptoms and do the things we can do until change is achieved.

Culture of Diagnosis and Judgment

One can discuss the culture of diagnosis and judgment which accompanies almost all human references endlessly. This phenomenon is so common that most people cannot distinguish the facts from the interpretation. Interpretation is perceived as an irrefutable fact. When people repeat the same judgment time and time again, it is perceived in their brain as a solid fact so that there is almost no chance that additional information will sink in and change their perception.

I see this as brain damage. It is caused as a result of the way our parents and teachers educated us and fed us, instead of providing us with the tools to think independently and prepare our brains to contain diversified scenery without locking each piece of information into a preconditioned and limited box of prejudice.

This culture causes many obstacles. Below I will discuss the main ones:

Inability

People who perform diagnosis tend to focus on a person's inabilities. So many people focus on the negatives (I do not know mathematics, I do not like children, I do not know how to sing etc.) and miss the positive things that they do (I do like to read, I do know how to cook, I do enjoy nature). People always look for the weaknesses and failures in themselves and in others. If you look hard enough, you will find an endless number of weaknesses in any person. This does not mean you have managed to diagnose this person's problems nor define his identity. It is as if you have looked everywhere but at the person himself. Some people mistakenly consider it a negative observation or criticism. It is not necessarily a negative observation but rather a lack thereof.

The Deterministic Element

Another obstacle could be when we refer to a single element of a person's ability separately from all his other abilities. In other words, we make a crude generalization – for better or for worse – based on a single element. For instance, a person who excels in one domain perceives himself as excellent in all domains and other people also perceive him as a person whose opinion matters in all other areas as well. Another could be, a singer who is interviewed regarding his political beliefs or a footballer who advertises a dairy product, or actors who express their opinions on relationships and parenthood and so forth.

Diagnosis based on symptoms is related to this subject as well. "Dyslexic," or "hyper-active" define a child's identity according to a specific symptom. The therapeutic culture urges us to pay special attention to symptoms. This phenomenon of defining according to symptoms is so rooted in our culture that we do not even doubt the processes of diagnostic thinking. Parents, teachers, psychologists, psychiatrists and so forth – they all make diagnoses. Most people focus on diagnosis and therefore readily accept the diagnostic verdict given to them, thus identifying with it. So many people introduce themselves to me by saying: "I am dyslexic," "I am asthmatic" as if these characteristics are written on their I.D. cards.

Structure of Personality

Crude diagnosis is the reason that most people perceive human beings as unchangeable. "A character does not change," "This is who I am," "It's genetic," "Parents determine our character," "We have a certain structure of personality" – these are examples of popular, common declarations. If we think of the term "Structure of Personality," it is a psychologist's concept which convinces us that we have a fixed personality, like buildings.

It's true that some things are unchangeable and we should not waste our time and energy on them; but we should not miss the things that **can** be changed. Similarly, a person who believes that parents have a great impact on the development of a child is like a person who repeats the first grade over and over again. Indeed, a person who keeps growing and developing is influenced by his parents to a certain extent, but he also learns from other people along the way and it is these interactions that can change his impressions of previous experiences. It would be a a pity to give up the chance to shape your own identity and therefore your own life because of common educational and psychological ignorance. A person who experiences the same things over and over again is not part of the scholastic culture but rather resembles a goat that grazes in the same pasture time and time again.

Diagnosis based on Sensations

Sensational diagnoses can be compared to shortsightedness. A person knows how he feels and believes that it reflects reality but he has no clue about the actual reality. The difference is that a shortsighted person knows that he does not see well. He finds ways to improve his sight, using glasses, a microscope, or a telescope. The sensational diagnostician does not attempt to improve his sight and understanding. On the contrary; he determinedly rejects whatever does not fit into his understanding or sensations.

We learn to sense and to feel, and if you wish, to think, in the same way we acquire our mother tongue language. Just like we cannot choose where to be born or what is fed into our brain. Thus, a person who diagnoses reality based on how he feels at a certain moment **only** reflects the elements he has accumulated so far and misses the opportunity to learn new things. People who say: "It feels right," or "It feels wrong," remain with the same old experiences, reaching the same conclusions and making the same judges over and over again. Therefore, therapy based on discussions of feelings, emotions, "what does it do to you" and the like only encourages people to remain in the same grade and to recycle themselves instead of growing and developing. In my opinion, if a person is disgusted by a certain food, it does not mean that the food is not tasty. In most cases, it is an expression of the person's previous experiences and his/her unwillingness to learn and to develop his/her ability to enjoy new types of foods.

Nevertheless, almost everyone can, with a certain amount of effort, identify within his reservoir of experiences, certain feelings that have changed completely. For instance, a person who once did not like a certain type of music can learn, in time, to enjoy it, once he is afforded the opportunity to enjoy it and change his attitude. In "Friendship School" we do not sit idly by and wait for the mere chance to ignite the process of change.

The fact that our emotions and feelings are not necessarily untrue complicates things even further. In fact, there is no limit to our learning efforts. We must consistently sharpen our learning tools, catch-up, learn our lessons, better the things that need to be improved and ask ourselves – What should we add to our life so that we will have a relatively reliable tool to find our way in the world? In short, in "Friendship School" we do not focus on the things a person feels like doing, but rather on the things that are worthwhile doing.

Shaping Identity, Change

Dealing with the question – 'what is in the best interest of a person?' – is fascinating. It involves getting to know each person and referring to him personally and accurately. Since the things that are important for one person might be completely irrelevant as far as another person is concerned.

The experience and overall viewpoint of scholastic people does not allow for crude diagnosis. A scholastic person knows that he can never see all the elements of the situation. He is constantly on the move and sees all shades of the circumstances, according to his personal point of view. He knows his limits and does not assume his judgments are definitively correct. So, instead of restricting himself and his environment within a predetermined pattern, he maintains a sense of curiosity and a desire for learning that enables him to consistently acquire new information. Each additional piece of information changes his previous understanding and interpretation while at the same time, changes him.

Change is produced by adding a new ability to a person's existing reservoir of abilities. It is <u>the</u> additional ability that changes the person's identity. Learning to drive, for example, changes a person's identity from a pedestrian to a driver. Producing the friendly change is created through production and management. Metaphorically speaking, we plant the actions and deeds we consider necessary for producing change in our garden-beds. The question – What should we invest in? – is a personal one. Each person is supposed to realize what is in his best interest and then invest in promoting it. So, instead of philosophizing about change, we promote it from day to day. As said before, in "Friendship School" we bypass the symptom and concentrate all our efforts on promoting the desired ability, which does not necessarily have to be related to the symptom. For instance, the homework given to spouses who fight endlessly is to learn Salsa and to try new positions during sex. However, even if the homework is directly related to the symptom we do not deal with appeasement but rather on promoting ability. When dealing with examination anxiety, for example, we add mini-situations which contain all sorts of constraints to the ability of answering questions, at home, under optimal conditions. The constraints might range from the need to provide quick answers to the presence of an audience – until the examinee acquires the ability to express his knowledge during high-pressure and stressful situations. We would deal with a singer who suffers from stage-fright in a similar manner. Such a person should add to his singing ability the ability to entertain people. He/she should sing occasionally for a small audience whilst gradually gaining confidence and developing his entertainment ability, which would have previously caused him/her must stress. The performer should continue doing this until accustomed to performing in front of a bigger audience. A similar thing happens when we move from an individual sexual expression such as masturbation, to a sexual expression which involves another person.

If someone feels the same things over and over again, and they deal with similar experiences in the same manner, it means that true learning has not taken place. <u>True learning really changes the way we feel.</u>

An Island of Ability

Learning is not all about homework. The most important element of learning and producing change is not merely about doing – but involves a certain type of **concentration** on what we do. Just as holding a book and looking at the lines is not exactly reading. What turns it into reading is the concentration and the subsequent effort to understand the written words.

A comment about concentration: students at the "Friendship School" do a great deal of homework in order to improve their ability to concentrate and develop thinking skills. We can compare it to the ability to control the movement of our head and the look in our eyes. A person whose sight and neck muscles are functioning is capable of turning his head freely and staring at whatever he chooses. One can acquire freedom of thinking, which enables a person to concentrate on whatever he chooses, in a similar way. This ability can be assimilated through practice.

In "Friendship School" we use this skill extensively. What should we concentrate on? This is a crucial element of learning. Most people focus on expected feelings such as anxiety, disgust and difficulty, and keep focusing on the negative aspects or expectations of oneself.

Scholastic people refer to this expectation as if it were a distracting noise and focus on <u>actually</u> growing and developing ability. They concentrate on the flavor of the food and not on the pre-programmed sense of disgust. They focus on the kiss and not on being stressed out by the presence of a woman. They concentrate on the new words being added to the language

Instead of looking at the sea of inabilities surrounding us we choose to focus on the island of abilities, which expands and enhances our identity, shaping it according to our own personal choice.

A person who focuses on the above knows that change is taking place. The scope of change will depend on the scope of his/her investment. This is the most optimistic and friendly fact and this is what I offer my students. <u>This can also be considered the weak point of the method</u>. It is based on a determined scholastic culture. A person who doesn't make an effort to learn and who isn't persistent in his efforts will remain the same. The therapist does not have any enforcement tools to enforce change. The high rate of success in "Friendship School" is mainly linked to the fact that I simply dismiss the learning decliners.

Most people prefer a supportive treatment that on the surface appears as if the person is really doing something in order to change, without really changing at all.

Method's Application

Friendship is an art that has to be acquired and nurtured. It is an essential ability which is at the basis of success in most areas of life; professional and social. This is an "obligatory" subject – since things that are related to individuals require learning and reference to people, whether it is about spouses, parents and children or business partners.

Some people acquire this <u>art</u> in their first learning environment; at home - if they were lucky enough to be raised by people who had learnt how to enjoy each other. People who were not that lucky must make the conscious decision to develop the 'friendly' ability. This method of acquiring the "friendship ability" applies to various life situations These include:

Singles

Most single people are egocentric. They do not know how to take another person into consideration and thus seek someone who is willing to adapt to their limitations or expectations and their search is often fruitless. They only give their date a chance when they sense a "click" or certain "chemistry on the first date. In most cases, the following dates greatly disappoint them. In "Friendship School" a match is the result of a lasting friendship between two individuals who have become experts on one another. Students conduct a set of guided dates; this is neither match-making nor a commitment for life. It is simply a commitment to hold a number of meetings in which each person is supposed to be at their best. They do their homework together: <u>she is his homework and he is her homework</u>. Following each meeting, each person writes a report in which they specify the things they have learnt about the other person and add recommendations in order to progress even further in the next meeting.

Both people bring with them a package of abilities that they have acquired prior to meeting each other. A person who knows how to seize an opportunity relates to the other's abilities. They each take even the smallest portion of what is offered by the other person, essentially killing two birds with one stone. His world is expanded and enriched by the things he has learnt from the other person. He also allows himself to enjoy the company of the other person and lets it enrich his development.

When two strangers come from the scholastic culture, their relationship develops constantly and becomes more interesting and rewarding.

This method is extremely efficient. Sometimes, people who started seeing each other as "homework" became a couple that continued to grow together. Dating, however, does not always necessarily have to lead to that result. It also happens that, after a while, people feel that they have nothing else to gain from the relationship and choose to develop further with other partners.

When two people decide to become a couple, it is not merely a matter of living together, but an identity change. A person who becomes a friend, a husband or a father, and believes he does not have to change in any way, is wrong. In order to become a spouse who is also a friend, one must change, because his identity now includes another person. The place the other person now occupies in his world does not allow him to maintain his previous identity just as one cannot go back to kindergarten after graduating from high school. Needless to say, this is not an isolated step; it is a process that is supposed to last. Once we stop learning how to be a couple, we are stuck; the same would have happened if we had stopped practicing the piano. Over some time, our previous ability fades away and if we wish to regain this ability, we must start practicing again.

Couples

It is not easy to maintain a long-term relationship, especially in a world where social contacts and media offer a great deal of temptation and opportunities. Nevertheless, many people manage to survive as a couple for many years. The main reason for this is that most spouses believe in the notion of belonging to each other. They exist side by side for many years, like pieces of furniture.

In other words, it is a connection between two committed people who are content with little and remain confined within a relationship. From time to time, an "accident" occurs – one of the spouses becomes involved with another person and the unit is 'broken'. A relationship that is not nurtured constantly, is a neglected relationship, which ultimately results in "accidents." In most cases the "accidents" are romantic entanglements in the workplace or in social circles to which only one of the spouses belongs.

The notion that once two people get married, they no longer have to court each other is totally incorrect. Spouses who do not know how to maintain the romance and excitement in their marriage are doomed to fail, or to settle for a limited relationship. Very few people know how to maintain an enthralling relationship filled with laughter, one that is full of satisfaction and mutual expression and respect that continues to develop throughout the years. Such a relationship is very hard to compete with.

It is also not easy to produce change in a relationship. The commitment binds each of the spouses to their previous habits. The spouse's treaty resents the therapist determinedly.

On the contrary, if both spouses belong to the scholastic culture, it is very easy to produce change. For instance, it is much easier to lose weight as a couple. It is much easier to learn something new when you are accountable to another person.

There is no point in diagnosing a relationship since traditional psychology is not capable of identifying so many diverse and complicated situations, which contain so many versions and combinations. Thus, in the "Friendship School," we do not focus on the things that ostensibly cause certain problems between the spouses; we do not make room for a celebration of complaints and arguments, since by doing so we only encourage the couple to keep using the same language, instead, we immediately consider the things which are worthwhile for the spouses individually and together.

If two spouses make the conscious decision to invest in promoting their relationship, change will easily be achieved: this means that they are both committed to investing in the quality of their relationship, open to innovative ways to perpetuate this quality.

It should be noted that an upgrade or advancement in the relationship is also needed when a couple wishes to produce a desirable change in their adolescent children.

If the spouses do not engage in development together, the one that agrees to become part of the scholastic culture will change independently. Sometime his/her change provokes and motivates the other spouse to change as well. If there continue to be gaps or divisions between the spouses, the one who keeps developing has a chance to produce change in the relationship, if he/she can overcome the challenges of change. In other words, this spouse should be daring enough to disturb the balance in the relationship and to be considered "wrong" in order to promote the necessary change. For example, if a man becomes depressed after being fired from his job, his family will have to adjust to his mood, feeling as though they have to walk on egg shells when they are around him to avoid upsetting him further. His wife eventually goes out without him and starts living a full, rewarding life: she works, she goes out, she takes care of the children, she does not need his help and she acts as if she were a single mother. Her behavior might motivate her husband. In this relationship, the wife has actively changed and therefore influenced the nature of the relationship. If the husband makes the decision to change accordingly, they would move forward together. If he remains unchanged, he may lose his spouse. The person who produces the initial change is the capable partner in the relationship. I consider this approach a friendly one since it creates change in the 'sick' partner more efficiently than all existing psychological and psychiatric treatments. If the 'sick' partner does not get better, at least the capable partner and other members of the family are free to change their destiny. In "Friendship School" quarrels are considered a popular pastime among people who are not smart enough to think of a more interesting form of entertainment. We do not focus on the nature of the quarrels, but rather on their frequency. Spouses, who know how to have a good time together, would prefer to enjoy each other's company than fight all the time. The solution to frequent quarrelling is two-fold: for change decliners – segregation and minimization of the relationship – and for those interested in change, investing attention during the time spent together, which may increase their ability to enjoy each other's company and reduce the frequency of quarrels.

Friendship with Children

Parenthood has become an impossible profession. Parents are expected to follow endless instructions from medical and psychological "administrators." Most people believe that the sooner they pay attention to problematic symptoms the better. When parents anticipate a child's failures instead of focusing on his developing abilities; they shape his identity as one who has a problem, therefore damaging his development. Young children perceive themselves through the eyes of adults. Any kindergarten teacher can send a mother for a set of checkups at various institutions. Pre-emptively diagnosing a child can be a felonious act. Their independent learning ability is wondrous and in the scholastic culture it is easy to expand on the abilities of a child. Instead of promoting this development, many adults repress and castigate the child. In many places around the world children are put into an educational production line that is intended to subjugate the child for the sake of a state, a religion or a terrorist organization. In most cases it succeeds and it is if the child's brain and freedom of thought is eliminated. The child eventually follows the path laid out for him by his parents and teachers and from this point on he simply acts and behaves predictably, like so many other animals in nature.

I resent the idea of putting blame on children. In the "Friendship School" there is no point in discussing the children outside of their culture of family context. The parents are the ones who create the family's language, and children are the byproduct of this language. Similarly, there is no point blaming children in Budapest for speaking Hungarian. Children react to whatever they sense is preoccupying their parents and obey the cultural standards their parents set. Sometimes they resent their parents' repression (some children give up on the chance of being accepted by their parents and act out **against** the system. There are many phenomena which can be seen as a type of protest – the child is willing to sacrifice his identity in order not to be repressed by his/her parents or dominant adults in his/her life. In any case, young children do not live in a vacuum. First, you should <u>nurture your relationship</u> with your spouse. This is the most worthwhile investment as far as you and your children are concerned. Nevertheless, friendship with children is not that complicated and would be a pity to miss. The best foundation to children's growth is the friendship between the spouses. They notice how much mother enjoys father and father enjoys mother, so go for it. Secondly, <u>invest in yourself</u> and develop your ability to enjoy all kinds of activities. It does not require money and investments but brains and culture. Ride your bike, sing. You can enjoy singing even if you do not sing like a professional singer. Dance, fly kites, go to the beach, travel, laugh, bake cakes and so forth.

Invite your children to do these activities with you. You do not have to do things which bore you. Your children will notice that. The most essential thing is that parents release themselves from their egocentric hoops in the presence of their children. In other words, <u>be at your best</u> in front of your children. Most parents have this ability and they are indeed at their best at work and in the presence of people who are important to them. They are now asked to use this ability in the presence of their children as well.

The most important principal is to not serve your children, but to rather serve their development. This means that you are supposed to let your baby hold his/her bottle initially, and later on his spoon, thus enabling him/her to feed him/herself. In other words, you should prefer promoting his/her ability in ensuring the cleanliness of the house. This is not a permanent situation. The child's ability develops as quickly as lightning and it should soon enable him to eat without making a mess at all. Additionally, you should also teach your child to take you and his/her siblings into consideration. The more his capacity for consideration develops, the more it enables him to participate in your cultural pastimes.

Let me elaborate a little. 'Friendly' parents are aware of their exact abilities as well as their limitations and do not present themselves as omnipotent. For instance, I know absolutely nothing about electronics and computers. My children are aware of this limitations and do not expect me to help them or share knowledge with them in this regard. I, however, respect their expertise in this field and derive pleasure from their abilities. They are aware of my other abilities and skills and respect me in those areas and in that regard.

'Friendly' parents notice the fast growing abilities of their children. They enable their children to enjoy their parents' abilities and include them in the activities they like to participate in and what they are good at. These children will meet their parents where they are at their best. This encourages the children to be at their best as well. In such a way, it is possible to avoid a static crude pattern of parenthood. A six year old child might have a specific superior ability compared to his parents – for example, an ability related to computers. At the age of ten he might swim better than his parents and excel in other areas as well –but still be able to enjoy spending time with them. The parents are supposed to teach him to take them and his siblings into consideration. This way, the child gets to know various social combinations, which will widen his horizons and enrich his emotional experiences. He will know how to conduct himself when he is by himself and when there are other people around.

As long as he is incapable of taking others into consideration, he will not be invited or included in group activities. Therefore, he will develop a sense of longing to develop social skills as it will open new, interesting doors for him. When we do not include our child, we are not necessarily punishing him. Punishments force parents to act like police officers and promotes negative interactions. Not taking the child is essentially about reconciling between his abilities and the reality. An adult cannot enter an event without the appropriate ticket. It should be the same with our children. We should not let them join a trip if they do not have the ability to be considerate to other participants. A baby can spoil the enjoyment of the whole family. It is not friendly. We teach him/her something which is irrelevant outside of the family dynamic.

I resent the contemporary trend of restoration when looking at parental authority. It reminds me of slogans such as 'relive your past' or 'honor thy father and thy mother'. This is a crude approach which is typical of a militaristic, short-sighted and narrow-minded type of thinking. We, the parents, should show the savage who runs the show. A more broad-minded person understands that most children will abandon their studies and all other activities which are forced upon them the minute they have the chance to do so. Moreover, some of them will react to their parents the same way should they attempt to make their lives miserable. Even if the child develops burdensome behavior patterns it is not advisable to drag him to psychological treatments. His parents, having received short guidance, should produce more change in him than any psychologist could.

Friendship with Adolescents

There is a myth regarding adolescents which suggests that they must experience a serious crisis called the "adolescence crisis." Children whose parents are growth and change decliners, grow and subsequently reach the ceiling that their parents put above their heads. Some adolescents do not develop further and remain "good children" in the negative sense of the word – namely, they are obedient and programmed limited as their parents would want them to be. They do not enjoy personal freedom to explore the world. Neither the parents nor the adolescents can truly be satisfied with this.

Other adolescents develop further out of crude rebellion against their parents. Their path is full of obstacles and bitter struggles. While there are certain advantages to this developement, the costs are sometimes high as often mental resources are wasted. Parents who avoid the fact that their adolescent has an independent ability, and insist on crude and limiting parenthood, might push their adolescent into risky places. On the other hand, parents in the scholastic culture enable their adolescents to continue with the process of growth and their subsequent production of abilities.

'Friendly' parents derive much benefit from their children's growth, which enables them to "resign" from their full - time job as parents. They take advantage of the free time and use it to enrich their own relationship and promote their cultural development whilst still learning something from their adolescents. In other words, instead of judging the adolescents, often unfavorably, parents are supposed to grab the opportunity and rather learn from their adolescents. In this way, the parents can enrich their own identity, relate to contemporary culture and equip themselves for future developments which may knock on their door. Thus, they derive much more satisfaction from their life and are able to maintain a friendly relationship with their adolescents. Other parents are left behind and do not understand the world around them: they are stuck in the same place, in a world they consider the best, and see the "new" world as a distorted one. Needless to say, this situation leads to wide gaps occurring between parents and children.

It is important that adolescents equip themselves with the ability to sift through the various possibilities that they are confronted with and find their own way in the world. A person whose thinking tools are rudimentary cannot handle his energies and the numerous prospects he may come across. He is not patient enough to develop his identity and he needs immediate, crude solutions. It is typical of penitents who believe in decisive solutions and clear vision. It is also typical of zealous fans of sports teams and members of gangs. On the other hand, those who are equipped with friendlier thinking tools will experience an adolescence period which is rich in experiences that are fascinating and enriching and will therefore not need to use unfriendly, destructive means.

Psychosomatics

Spending time focusing on potential illnesses resembles any other kind of pastime. Moreover, it might even be more addictive. Contrary to popular opinion, I believe it is much easier to suffer than to enjoy life. In order to develop an ability to enjoy, we must actually invest in it, but a relief derived from feelings of suffering and pain is available to all and easily achieved. Until one reaches the point where he enjoys his piano playing he must make consistent effort and, on the other hand, spending time in medical examinations and treating illnesses is now much more readily available. Thus, I believe that a person who wishes to develop a healthy identity must decide to be part of the scholastic culture.

In addition, a person who does not feel well and diagnoses his physical condition as a fragile one, is expected to become sick in time. Stomach aches might turn into an ulcer, heart sensitivity might turn into a heart disease and so forth. Just as a person who practices the piano consistently eventually becomes a pianist, a person who is always occupied with diseases develops the identity of a sick person. Fortunately, only very few people are doomed to be sick, injured and/or seriously limited. Most patients choose to be overly occupied with diseases in their free time.

Even if someone is really suffering from a chronic disease or a certain deformity, it does not necessarily mean his identity should be one of a sick or disabled person. Let's take for example a person who has become blind. Obviously he cannot see. Many people would build their whole identity based on this limitation and develop the identity of a disabled person for life and pertaining to all areas of life. But such a person could also choose to develop his identity as a musician, a writer, a teacher, a spouse, a parent and so forth. In other words, such a person can combine his limitation with the other components of his identity. When I meet such a person I have to remind myself he cannot see, since this person puts his identity ahead of his disability – his abilities rather than his limitations.

Professional Identity

Instead of trying to find yourself, in "Friendship School" we suggest learning how to shape your identity. Before we deal with big, central questions such as "What will you be when you grow up?" or "What, in your opinion, will make you a satisfied, happy person"? We create and develop the tools that enable us, with time, to deal with the bigger questions. As a first step each one of us should start shaping the next morning. The next evening. To invest in certain types of management that would make Sunday more interesting, more entertaining. In other words, focus on building a personal operating system of time management. It is not just about passing time by watching T.V or passing time with a few other bored people at a bar, but rather about engaging in activities that could enrich your or other people's abilities.

If a person still does not succeed in enjoying or making the best of his personal time, he should not mislead himself into thinking that he will succeed in producing a set of complex related activities that will lead to changing his identity. (Nevertheless, we should not forget that many people around the world do not even reach the point where they deal with identity questions. They are born into certain pre-planned targets and their whole daily schedule is dedicated to reaching these targets. The best example is people who are born into certain religious communities).

While doing his homework within the scholastic culture framework, the client's time fills up with all sorts of interesting, beneficial activities and soon his world includes all sorts of hobbies. A certain part of the day is dedicated to providing a particular service and getting paid for it. When a person develops his ability related to this service, he, in fact, builds the infrastructure that will enable him to develop a professional capability and an expertise that will become a more central part of his identity. In time he discovers what should become his profession and what should remain a secondary pastime or a hobby; shaping his identity is based upon the amount of time he dedicates to each of the above activities. I, for instance, started dedicating more and more time to psychology and less and less time to my guitar practicing and other activities. This is why I became a psychologist who occasionally plays the guitar and sings. A different person could have become a guitar player and a singer who sees psychology as a hobby. In the scholastic culture almost everybody can discover within himself a wide variety of ability segments and fragments of talents which might cause confusion and hesitation. Moreover, we cannot possibly take advantage of the numerous possibilities surrounding us. There are far more books than we can ever possibly read, more men and women than we can possibly love and so forth. That is the reason why it is highly important that we develop our ability to sift through and select from all the possibilities the one that would best reflect our talents. A person who has learnt how to do that enjoys his activities and lives the most satisfactory life. He shapes his identity based on his best ability and not on his limitations.

Friendship in Businesses and Organizations

Instead of dealing with problems, in the "Friendship School" we deal with promoting the interests of the business or organization. First, we find the capable people, the ones who are friends of the institution, the ones who are capable of sensing the things that might promote their work place and the interests of their employees. These people should have more senior roles. The shaping of their roles should be done according to the variety of their abilities. People should learn about each other's abilities and enjoy what each person has to offer. Capable people should take responsibility for new employees or more limited employees and make sure their work bears fruit. They are supposed to identify people who have an ability to learn and who might become friends of the institution in the future. The several people who cannot be friends of the institutions, who are not capable of learning and changing, who constitute a burden and damage the institution should be dismissed or put into harmless positions.

When we know how to take advantage of people's talents outside the workplace, and produce entertaining and cultural channels of expression out of the reservoir of employees – the workplace, what was once just a source of income, becomes a pleasant place. We might as well enjoy the activity we dedicate most of our time to; since most people spend more time at work than at home.

Creative Thinking

Most thinking people use the tools of analysis and logic; namely, they analyze a situation based on a certain analytic tool and reach conclusions derived from their analysis. Others don't even think, but make do with reciting out of their existing reservoir of understanding stemming from their primary education. This process makes their way of thinking a fixated, predictable one. If they come across a thought which does not match their opinion, they usually use their rejection reflex – and rely on the same bunch of opinions, already planted in their brains. Even if they come up with a certain innovative idea, they immediately "kill" it with a contradicting one.

In 'friendly' thinking we do not reject any ideas but rather add them to the reservoir of ideas. Therefore, all ideas and thoughts are placed side by side and it is possible to scan them without reflexes of diagnosis, pre-judgment or rejection. In the scholastic culture, curiosity knows no limit; freedom of thought is endless and all sorts of "truths" are not taken for granted. Thus, the scenery in front of us becomes more extensive and one can discover in it many more combinations and possibilities compared to the landscape of the narrow-minded person. Eventually, choosing the combination which seems best to us drives away all other possibilities. When a person practices this type of thinking and nurtures it, an infrastructure is created and serves as the basis of revelations that are innovative and creative.

Politics

It is not easy to define a person and characterize him based on a crude diagnosis. It is not easy to assume his best interests. It is far more difficult to diagnose couples and families and promote their interests. Diagnosing nations and countries, knowing what their best interests are and promoting them is truly an impossible task.

In elections, most people vote based on an automatic reflex, which is far from being based on reasoning and certainly not on 'friendly' reasoning. Even people who believe that they base their vote on well-argued reasoning do not see how predictable and fixated their opinion is. Most votes are traditional and predetermined.

Most politicians do not perceive themselves as people who serve the public and promote their best interests. They are mainly concerned with encouraging their voters to keep on voting for them. They do not invest in education which promotes abilities related to thinking, selecting and growing, since it will force them to be more developed and enlightened than they usually are. They are narrow-minded clerks. Even a child in the third grade can lead a herd of second-grade children, and as long as they are willing to remain in a lower grade, the leader can afford to remain as is.

Nevertheless, our world is constantly changing, and the speed of change is not always easy to follow. In the past, the planet was so big that each nation was separated from other nations and there was no friction. Nowadays, our world is so crowded that referring separately to national or religious perception might damage the national interest since it often does not take the outside world into account. Just like a team player who plays as if he were by himself instead of joining forces with the rest of the players, for the sake of the team. If the team fails, he too will be one of the losers.

Nurturing and teaching values is not especially efficient. All religions call for the love of mankind, and still, throughout the generations, religion was the main cause of bloodshed. Values are pointless unless they are accompanied by the ability to accept people who are different than us, the ability to become friends with them. A person, who is not capable of that, is forced to reject and hate people who do not fit into his narrow world. Spouses who do not know how to be friends fight a lot. When members of different religions and nations come across each other and they are not equipped with the ability to make friends, it turns into bloodshed. Nowadays, many nations own weapons which are capable of blowing up entire continents, therefore, promoting the ability to make friends is essential to the survival of humankind.

So far I have described the gist of the method. For further information please refer to my other books and/or the friendly lexicon which can be found on our internet site. You are also invited to join one of the courses in "Friendship School."

Introduction
Everyone Can Change

Yes, everyone can change.

I, for example, went through a significant change. I was born and raised as a religious boy, and here I am today, completely secular. To a great extent I shaped my new identity. Even professionally I went through a significant change. I used to be a clinical psychologist. Then I retired from traditional psychology and created a new system I called "The Friendship School," through which I accompany many others who are going through the process of change. I believe my personal experience enables me to help others find the appropriate means to make friendly changes themselves.

This book presents the ways that, according to my experience, lead to change. The bulk of the technology of change (yes, even when talking about emotional change, there is room for the word "technology") was developed and formulated over many years, partly due to the lessons I learned from my own successes as well as my failures, which were plentiful. The guidelines for change have been refined again and again, purified in the crucible of life, leading to considerable successes. In other words, my theory has evolved from experience.

I started by saying that everyone can change, yet most people do not go through major changes in their lives. Why is that? After decades of work with a great variety of people in different situations, I believe that change happens to those who make a special effort to bring it about. Few people are aware of the great contribution change can make in improving our lives and maximizing pleasure and satisfaction. Those who are not aware of this have a hard time achieving change. The tools I will present here enable us to learn the friendly paths that lead to change. Nevertheless, understanding these methods is not enough. One needs to practice. Whether you choose to walk down one of the paths, or not, depends first and foremost on you.

I say "paths," in the plural, since I am not proposing a single method or one clear-cut course on the map of a personal journey. I believe there is no "right" or "wrong" path, and each of us has his or her own personal path. The milestones mentioned in this book form a mosaic, combining to create a whole picture: for each his own. I am certain that almost every reader who finishes reading this book can pave a path suitable for him or herself

The saying that 'there is no justice in the world' can be said about change. Just as some of us are born with silver spoons in our mouths, others have to struggle to reach a reasonable financial situation, this is the case here too. Some are equipped with outstanding means for change. They need only pick them up and use them. Others need to take pains to invent these means. For them, change is not an easy task. Those of us raised with firm "dos" and "don'ts" and clear "rights" and "wrongs" have to make a special effort to bring about change, if we so wish.

This book has three parts. The first part discusses change and its significance. The chapters in the second part focus on the implementation of change in different fields of life. Last but not least, the third part discusses the process of change from two angles – that of the psychologist (the guide to change) and that of the client (I do not like the term patient). The book begins with a glossary of terms which includes brief explanations of my conceptual terminology. I recommend using the glossary constantly throughout the reading of the book.

Before beginning, here is some friendly advice.

To browsers: do not hurry to find the chapter dealing with the particular issue that is bothering you personally. You never know when new insights may dawn. Learning may well happen when you are exposed to a topic that does not affect you personally.

And to everyone: in many of the chapters, there are some practical exercises. These are necessary for producing change and for the creation of a new identity, since to succeed on the road ahead, we must practice again and again the skills we have not yet developed. Some of the exercises in the book should be practiced dozens of times a day. Some are vital in laying a good foundation for learning and for sharpening the tools needed along the way. Others will help us when we are in a particular bind. It is important to note that even the exercises included in chapters dealing with specific issues are relevant to the whole process of change. Such, for example, is the exercise that helps us focus our sense perception. Though it is included in the chapter dealing with changes in our sex lives, it is central to every aspect of our lives.

The book contains many examples taken from real life. Despite the significance of the examples, you must not allow them to distract from the essence. You should avoid an absolute identification with particular examples ("This is exactly how it is for me!"), and an exact replication of the conclusions and the methods described in an example. Likewise, you should try not to parry an example with scorn if it has nothing to do with you. ("Why, the example deals with a woman, whereas I am a man, and a redhead at that!") Either reaction precludes learning. The examples are important thought exercises, in which the search for one's own path is more important than the conclusion.

Another comment, actually an apology. I feel the need to attack different psychological approaches. This is because these approaches are well-anchored in the media and academia, who market these wares as if they are unchallenged truths. Most people abide by these so-called truths, but I see it as my obligation to share with you, from the wealth of my experience, the understanding that some of these are mistaken and misleading. Naturally, my criticism is general and inclusive since I do not know all psychologists and psychiatrists personally. I am sure that many of their approaches lead to friendly change, and it does not matter which method they employ. Hence, we should always examine the particular case of each meeting with such a professional, while taking into account the actual benefits resulting from it. By benefits, I mean measurable ones that can easily be recognized, rather than vague feelings of improvement.

Actually, this is true not only in reference to canonical psychology. Throughout our lives, and before every decision we make, we should beware of purportedly "tested' advice. We should examine each particular case on its own merit. The same applies to the numerous suggestions appearing on the pages of this book. For instance, I repeatedly suggest, in a number of places in this book, that the single man or woman should date a number of people at once. This suggestion is right in some cases, and even many cases, but sometimes this advice – though I give it myself – is inappropriate. I remember a young woman who openly dated a number of men concurrently after reading one of my previous books, missing the chance to connect with a man who wished to spend all his free time with her, who was committed and was capable of true companionship. Another young woman accepted the advice I gave her – to dedicate a number of dates to each possible partner and not hurry to exclude anyone – too faithfully. She failed to notice the problems which arose in her dates with a particular man, which were of the type one should not ignore when building a relationship.

But bear in mind, dear reader, that I am sitting in front of my computer writing, while you are the subject. So, for every recommendation given here, you should ask yourself whether it is really appropriate for your particular situation. Continue to examine all suggestions you receive in a specific case, even after you finish reading this book.

To conclude, one last comment about language. The English language distinguishes between men and women, and attention to both sometimes demands cumbersome and clumsy wording. Therefore I choose sometimes to direct my words towards men or women only. Yet every recommendation, explanation or example is aimed at both sexes, depending on the context of course. So, for example, every mention of a boyfriend applies to a girlfriend as well, and vice versa.

Part 1

Chapter 1

Towards Change – The Friendly Change

Who needs a book about change?

Some people know how to grow and evolve continually, and when in trouble, creative solutions sprout within them. Those people are good-natured. They allow their loved ones to enjoy their abilities and are also able to enjoy others' successes. For them, it is a natural ability. They are bestowed with intelligence and a variety of talents, and they employ their abilities to achieve whatever goal they choose. Those people can do without this book.

Unfortunately most of us are not members of that group but belong to a second, much larger group. The members of this group have excellent abilities but miss out on something in life. It is as if something in their minds prevents them from realizing their potential, forces them to limit their aspirations, and condemns them to spend precious time on bothersome and unsatisfying concerns and tread water in relentless anguish. For many, their lives pass by in dejection and with a lack of satisfaction with themselves and the world. Others are satisfied with the way they run their lives, but in actuality they settle for less and miss out on the opportunity to live a much fuller life.

It is for the members of this group – those who are interested in succeeding in life and making the best of themselves – that this book is intended.

Who is ready for change?

Age is relevant to the ability to change. Everyone knows that a young immigrant child learns the language of his new home rather quickly and needs relatively few resources to learn what is necessary to acclimatize to his new surroundings. An adult immigrant, on the other hand, makes greater effort with fewer results. Thus it is no wonder that the majority of adult immigrants abandon the attempt to acclimate and prefer consorting with other immigrants from the same country in a kind of cultural ghetto.

And yet, the acceptable view according to which the old cannot change is mistaken. **The potential for change persists throughout the life cycle**. People who are accustomed to what I call a culture of learning as an integral part of life continue to learn and evolve until old age. Those not so accustomed will have a hard time making changes in old age. Yet this does not mean that adults and seniors who are strangers to the learning culture should give up. They should, however, realize that in order to change, they may sometimes need to make an exceptional effort. Change itself will happen slowly, but if sought and genuinely pursued, it will happen.

For young people too, the road is not always paved. Some avoid change even when it is offered to them. They tend to argue and often automatically recoil from any effort to help them. Some young people respond to my suggestions with immediate defiance, but I am not disturbed, nor do I take it personally. It is likely that prior to seeing me, this young person was the victim of so much harassment and nagging that by now he has ceased to examine each suggestion and rejects all of them without thought. He no longer discriminates between ideas meant to maintain his obedient ways (or return him to them), and those aimed at giving him opportunities for a fascinating journey. To be ripe for change, one must be able to examine each suggestion on its merits rather than preemptively rejecting any new idea.

Age and character are not the only factors that might inhibit change. Some physical difficulties limit our abilities before we even begin. A blind man cannot paint, and a one-legged man cannot run. But they too can change their view of themselves and mold their identity according to ability rather than limitations. In choosing a profession, for example, the one-legged man, instead of seeing himself as disabled, should choose a profession that does not depend on his legs. His missing leg does not stop him from being a psychologist, a rehabilitative social worker, a philosopher or a writer.

In any case, change is not a simple or obvious process. I believe this fact in itself can stimulate the will to begin a process that will lead, eventually, to the longed-for change. It is worth noting at this point that we need not change everything all the time from the ground up. If we are accustomed to tying our shoelaces in a particular manner, there is no need to bother to change that. But if we like a particular style of music and despise another, perhaps we should develop our listening abilities so that we can, for example, enjoy music with our children.

Exercise: One small change

Change is a difficult task, but not impossible. We can all do it. In order to see this, one should try making a small change in a not-too-significant area that will quickly show results. We are like the man about to paint a canvas: he checks the paint first in an unobtrusive corner, and only after it is absorbed to his satisfaction does he paint the rest of the canvas.

One example is changing our attitude towards a particular food. If as adults we avoid avocado because as children we were forced to eat it, we should now attempt a little exercise and turn avocado into a tasty treat. We can do this with new recipes or with a conscious modification of our personal tastes. After we succeed in this, we may try a slightly more difficult change. Remember, becoming open to change requires us to randomly break even the most stubborn habits.

Who stops us from making changes?

Making a change is not an impossible task. Many other tasks we perform are harder. Nevertheless, most of us do not develop this ability at all. Why is that?

The simplest answer is the educational system. Granted the first school for babies happens to be parents, but they do the best they can for their children, even if not all parents are perfect. A bad educational system, however, is a real failure. Theoretically, a good teacher can contribute greatly to the development of a child and even fix what parents mess up. As matters stand, however, parents are required to fix the problems the educational system causes. It happens too easily that everybody – both parents and teachers– pounces on the small child, acting like partners in a conspiracy aimed to make him fit the "right" system: well-behaved with his parents, hardworking in school, obedient to his leaders and, in some cultures, a loyal subject to his God and a compliant servant of the representatives of God on earth.

No doubt these systems have much wrong with them, but before we begin blaming external factors for our inability to change, perhaps we should begin with an important internal factor – our brain.

Chapter 2

Your Brain as Your Friend

On the wonders of the brain

The brain is a wondrous organ, more so than the one can grasp. Yet, at the same time, the many bugs or defects in its programming may keep us from advancing and prevent us from growing.

Sometimes I wonder what came first: Was it long-term faulty education that neutered so many brains, stole from them the ability to think, and left them only with the ability to recycle and reconstruct, that is to continue to function as previously programmed? Or maybe our brain is preprogramed for substandard thought patterns and this, in fact, is the reason why our current educational processes subsist? I reckon our brain is responsible for much of our foolishness, even if it does so in good faith.

The brain is a mighty and complex organ. It controls many other organs and supervises countless functions with incredible success. Is anyone actually aware of what goes on inside his body? Does anyone know, for example, how his spleen is faring today? The spleen usually functions well, as do all the other organs, which is why we fail to pay attention to this function of the brain. What else can, like the brain, handle so many things at once? Generally, if we don't systematically destroy our health, inside and out, our bodies function as they should – all thanks to the brain. This is simply wondrous.

Nevertheless, there is something about the tyranny of the brain that should perhaps concern us. The brain directs not only the spleen, but our conscious actions and thoughts. It is rather comfortable for us to be unaware of how the brain accomplishes all that, so much so that we sometimes forget to be aware.

As early as in the stage of sense perception, the brain sifts through and chooses what to perceive, what to disregard and what to ignore. When I was in the military, we went on a night maneuver, without advance notice of the lessons to be learned. After we had walked a few miles, the commanding officers instructed us to lie quietly on the ground. A few minutes later, they asked us to tell them what we had heard. For the most part, when walking in the dark, each had focused on his thoughts and not on his surroundings. Upon hearing the question, however, each exercised his memory and recreated sounds that had reached his ears: a distant car, a howling jackal and other sounds of the night.

Afterwards we were again asked to lie still, except this time we were explicitly told to listen. Our range of hearing seemed to increase incredibly. We heard so much – squeaks, knocks, swishes – a variety of sounds and faint noises. We were asked to distinguish those sounds relevant to our mission, such as metal clinking, guns cocking, water swishing in containers, branches breaking, voices murmuring, and so on.

It seems that the first time the sounds reached our ears but stayed on the outside. The brain did not let them in. The second time, the brain allowed the sounds to enter, and so we could sort through them and extract the relevant sounds – in this case, those relevant to military operations. Someone else, a nature photographer for example, would have noticed other sounds.

A similar exercise was practiced regarding sight, this time during the day. Again we traveled for a few miles, after which we were asked to recount what we had seen. One of us described a tree, another described a bend in the path, not much more. We continued walking, this time cued to notice our surroundings. Now we saw all kinds of things: bushes, flowers, paths, an animal carcass, an anthill and the particular horizon at that spot. Here too, the brain first decided, in advance, what to see and what not to see, whereas in the second part of the exercise, we told it to employ our sight more carefully, and our whole vision changed.

Illusions of perception

The filters that the brain uses without our direction affect, without our being aware, what we see as solid facts.

Consider the following optical illusion. Which of the horizontal lines is longer?

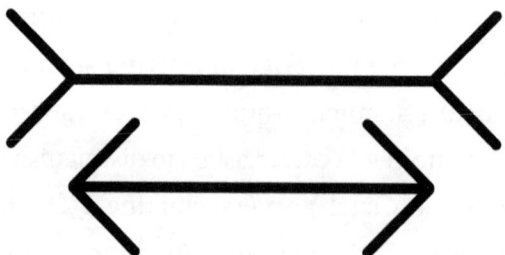

Actually, they are of equal length, and you are welcome to measure them. It is the outer lines that cause the optical illusion making one line seem longer than the other. Think therefore how easily one can "trick" this wondrous brain of ours. A few small lines, and the brain is misled. In that case, how can we trust it? How many other illusions affect us without our knowing it?

In a well-known experiment, students were asked to look at a picture while wearing lenses that had the effect of inverting what they saw. Normally, the retina receives an image upside down, and the brain's "corrections" are the reasons we see the image the way it is. Well, those students wore lenses that made everything seem upside down. For a while, these human guinea pigs were in a state of confusion and suffered from nauseating disorientation. After a few days of living with these lenses, their brains inverted the picture. Now, despite the lenses, they again saw reality normally. The experimenter – a sadist, it would seem – removed the lenses. The students again saw everything upside down and suffered from all the related side effects. Again, after a few days the picture "straightened," and they saw everything as usual.

These experiments show that the brain can affect our sense organs. Sometimes it does so because it *knows* what's right. At other times, as in the horizontal line case above, it is because it *thinks it knows* what's right.

Brainwashing

In ancient times, the world was, according to the scientists of the time, as flat as a pancake, since that is how the eye sees it. Later scientists discovered the world is as round as a ball, but were sure it was the center of the universe and the sun orbits it every day. Again, this is what the eye sees – every dawn the sun rises, and every evening it sets. The first who were brave enough to claim otherwise, that the earth orbits the sun like other planets, risked their lives. They were treated not only as weirdoes, but as criminals, and some of them were denounced and tortured by the Inquisition.

Different religious beliefs about the origins of the world, along with our understanding of sensory data, prevented us from seeing the truth. In general, the powers-that-be in the West refused to accept those who deviated from the norm. The Romans, for example, threw Christians into the lion's den but to no avail. A few hundred years later, amid the decline of the Roman Empire, Christianity became the dominant religion. The Christians, in turn, acted similarly: knowledge of the ancient world were destroyed in the name of religion. After the invention of the printing press, which enabled the dissemination of information circumventing the tyranny of the church, the latter continued to censor printed matter, burn books and execute revolutionary thinkers.

Religion is not solely responsible for brainwashing throughout history. Many a secular tyrant acted similarly. It suffices to mention Hitler and Stalin, who succeeded in brainwashing millions to kill or exterminate millions of other people of whom these dictators did not approve.

Actually, the ability to fool the brain has always been exploited by many. Here is a short list of such methods of exploitation: different potions sold by peddlers and soothsayers as remedies for incurable diseases; magical emulsions and love potions of various kinds; holy places, talismans and crystals; a profitable vitamin industry for the extension of life expectancy, hair growth and sexual potency;

astrology, which tells us our future based on Mars and Jupiter. These distortions are available in almost all media; and even by our elected politicians. Sometimes it seems that foolishness gets the best ratings. It is addictive. It is also hard to say which comes first: the calf yearning to suckle the milk of naïveté or the cow whose udders are filled with it.

Following years of research which involved tens of thousands of people, scientists tentatively concluded that exercise and a diet of fruit and vegetables are indeed beneficial to man, while everything else serves as a placebo. Generally, I am doubtful about such studies, as many of them are tendentious and serve various interests. I do not know why this particular study impressed me: perhaps because it agreed with what I thought beforehand based on my own experience, or perhaps because it was carried out in good faith. But perhaps I am mistaken. Perhaps the results of this study were biased in favor of the farmers' union.

By the way, placebos as such should not be disqualified out of hand, since many a time they achieve actual results. If the patient would know the medicine he's taking is nothing but flour in a capsule, perhaps mixed with a bit of dye, he wouldn't take it. Yet if he takes it, he does not benefit from the flour. So, we must ask, is the flour capsule beneficial or not? Of course not! But of course it is! On second thought, what is the significance of the answer to this question, so long as the patient, who was previously moaning with pain and could not sleep, is relieved after taking the placebo and can sleep? Granted, flour does not relieve pain. But our brain, that believes the pill is a pain reliever, is the factor which causes it to work.

Why do I argue against factors that so many believe are welcome and important? After all, religion and soothsayers often help those who believe, not unlike the placebo. Why is it then that I approve of placebos but not of different kinds of magical beliefs? My reason is that in the majority of cases, these beliefs replace the cultivation of our abilities. The strict believer does not ask what he himself can do. Rather, he conducts a ritual and hopes for the best. He thereby prevents himself from improving his life through learning and widening of his horizons. Obviously there are cases where belief does not harm ability. If the footballer runs like the wind, gives his all to the game and additionally carries a talisman in his pocket, it makes no difference. So be it.

I would like to take a little time here to deal with another factor that affects our brains and gets good ratings – anxiety. I find it hard to stand aside and see many unfriendly elements influence people as if they were automatons, weighing them down with mountains of worries. These elements succeed in doing so simply because their victims are obedient.

I believe that anxiety is a clumsy response to stimulus. Thinking critically about the stimulus would often enable us to see it in the right light. Consider for example the anthrax bacteria that does not not spread easily, so the chances of an epidemic are not high. If we place these bacteria on an open wound or the skin of someone who has recently showered, that person will catch the disease. Yes, make no mistake: scrubbing and wiping the skin leave minute scratches, making it more vulnerable to bacteria. And, if after that person catches the disease, no antibiotics are administered, he might even die. Nevertheless, the disease does not spread through air, and the risk of dying from it is lower than the risk of dying from another disease that does not stimulate public panic – the common flu.

Actually, when we so wish, we know exactly how to overcome anxiety. Consider driving. The risk of being killed as a result of a car accident is much higher than the risk of death from almost any other cause. Nevertheless, many of us travel from place to place without fear, and it wouldn't cross our minds to stop driving, just as we would not seriously decide to stop walking. We know there is a risk to driving, and that hardly a day goes by without someone dying on the roads. Nevertheless, we understand that the percentage of victims is small and the majority of drivers get home safely. We prefer therefore to focus on the abundant benefits of our increased mobility and drive carefully but not anxiously, and certainly without panicking.

Brain blocking

We are surrounded by constant stimuli. It is easy to permit entry to stimuli that suit our abilities and reject those that don't.

Those among us ready to learn, see stimuli as productive, something new that can stimulate curiosity. However, since certain stimuli may cause pain, many of us prefer to reject life's fluctuation towards pain. Others are reluctant to formulate wishes and desires for fear of disappointment. They opt for rejection of stimuli as a defense against pain. Some people live in a sort of cultural ghetto that prevents exposure to stimuli out of fear of the wish to break free.

Being blocked is like being in a confined hole, except that we are often unaware of it. In such situations we either live in monastic loneliness, or are surrounded by people who live like us, in the same limited world, who do not "threaten" to expose us to new things. We mostly feel good about this since there is virtually no divergence between our abilities and the world we are in. Perhaps the willingness to widen our horizons has not yet fully matured. We may believe that we control our world. We might actually feel better if we were to learn new things and evolve, but we are often not even aware of our limited horizons.

This kind of blocking is a solution for those of us who prefer a limiting and protective framework. But the arrangement has weaknesses. It is successful as long as we do not go beyond the boundaries of our chosen structure, as long as the borderline is solid and unbroken. When the boundaries are weakened or undermined, however, this "solution" becomes a problem. This may happen, for example, to a woman who decides to live alone, without room-mates or partners to spend time with, so she can dedicate herself to her studies. And yet, she lives in the big city and the sounds of life outside penetrate her ears. Occasionally she has times of quiet, when she is closed off in her apartment reading a book. But when she goes out, she sees couples embracing or finds out her schoolmate has gotten married and had a child. Her previously closed and protected world is violated. She needs to expend more and more energy to continue her limited existence, until eventually she fails to reach the original goal of dedicating herself to her studies.

Clearly, even the deliberate narrowing of our world takes time and energy. Consequently, our losses, and failiure to learn and evolve, outweigh the benefits.

Spiritual food or junk food?

Nowadays there's almost no point in trying to block the flow of information. Television, radio, internet and newspapers send the latest news from one side of the world to the other and reach every dark corner of the world. We are all aware that in totalitarian countries, tyrants still control the media and mold their citizens' lives according to narrow nationalist interests. But is television not a tyrant in democratic countries? And when it entertains the lazy brain and spreads folly in the name of ratings, is it not a complete waste? After all, this amazing medium could easily train the brain in ways that are both intelligent and entertaining and thereby enhance our thinking abilities rather than reducing them.

A similar question applies to our system of education. There is no doubt that in undemocratic countries the educational system is warped, teaching generations of students according to the interests of the ruling classes. But what about countries that brandish democracy as their flag? Does the education we and our children receive in such countries not serve the interests of certain groups more than we would like?

Distorted television and educational systems are two channels through which we feed our minds, and often we are unaware of the quality of the food. It may be in our interest to notice how we nourish our brains, just as we do concerning our bodies. We should ask ourselves about the quality of this nourishment. Are we providing our brains with food saturated with vitamins, food that will help the brain develop, or are we feeding it junk food that will simply give us the illusion of satiation? One can understand why the powerful elite would wish to restrict the minds of their subjects; because when the mind is free, the science-fiction of yesteryear becomes the acceptable science of today. Furthermore, the man whose mind is free may suddenly learn things that clash with conventional wisdom and may even disseminate his new found truths.

It is important, therefore, that we notice how we nourish our minds and control this as much as possible.

For a change – A wise investment in the brain

The brain stands at the root of the subject of this book – change. When dealing with change, it is best to dedicate oneself to the cultivation of the brain, since it is the organ in charge of forming identity. To make such an investment we should sharpen our learning gear. I am intentionally not referring to "thinking gear," in case someone concludes that it is enough to look towards the sky and meditate in order to initiate change or a friendly process. Bear in mind that not every high test score indicates an ability to think. Mostly, achievements are the result of repetition and memorization, and if we look into the brain of the high-achieving student we might find the usual mishmash of interpretation and facts.

It is therefore important to turn the brain into an instrument of learning. Without such an instrument, the learning process is slow and painful. However, once the brain knows how to learn, and we create a solution to one problem, solutions for many other problems will emerge as well.

This is analogous to playing an instrument. If I learn to read music and form chords, I will probably be able to accompany a song in no time. Yet if I only learn to play one particular song, I will only be able to accompany that song. If I then wish to accompany another song, I will have to learn the new song's chords. This is a Sisyphean effort. Each song requires a renewed effort, since I do not have the right foundation to accompany songs right away. Obviously, if I persist in learning song after song, I will learn to accompany new songs with increasing speed. However, this requires long and strenuous effort. If I learn how to form chords, however, my ability will develop faster and I may even acquire, in time, the ability to improvise. Who knows, I may even compose a song myself.

Accordingly we should, first and foremost, make the most of our abilities to think and learn. Developing these abilities, even if only in one area, affects other areas of our lives in a domino effect. A person with highly developed learning skills will treat his environment in a friendly manner and will consequently discover friendly and creative solutions to situations in which he would otherwise feel stuck.

In order to sharpen our learning tools we must cultivate in our brains the area of friendly thinking, which will, among other things, apply our existing abilities to new experiences. In other words: **instead of letting the brain lead us, we will lead it to new and exotic places**. We will use our brains for our own goals and relieve them of some of their damaging or counterproductive activities.

Cultivating friendly thinking

The area of friendly thinking, the type of thinking that can bypass the "automaticity" of the brain, will provide us with a starting point which we can use in areas of particular interest. Just as Archimedes claimed that if he had an external point of leverage he could lift up the whole world, we too are meant to find something outside our brains to act as leverage to work them harder.

If we fail to do so, the answers to our questions will be predictable. And we should know how to question ourselves, to ask, for example:

What is to my benefit? What can I do? What should I do? What new skills should I learn and how should I change my.....?

Some divide thinking into two types. One is magical thinking driven by feelings and beliefs. This type of thinking is not a good basis for any type of negotiation. Belief in itself is a type of thinking that bothers noone. The Amish, for example, lead their lives as they wish without it influencing those around them. The combination of faith with militaristic ability and money, on the other hand, can endanger the world. The Taliban is an example of such a lethal combination.

The other type of thinking acceptable as the "right" one in the Western world is logical-analytical thinking, which examines situations, derives conclusions and serves us all in all walks of life. This is the type of thinking learned in schools, and in my view it can be counterproductive. It does have its place and is beneficial in areas such as automotive or electrical engineering, where the analysis of a problem leads to the cause of the malfunction; merely knowing the cause enables one to reach a successful solution. And yet, when human beings are involved, those who act only according to such thinking miss out on a lot.

There is, however, a third type of thinking, namely friendly thinking. This type of thinking bypasses the limitations of logical-analytical thinking, producing endless prospects from which many scripts can be written, leading to incalculable paths and enabling free choice. This type of thinking is different from magical thinking in requiring the recognition of opportunities and acquisition of new abilities, hence contributing to our continual progress. It is worth noting that friendly thinking allows both logical-analytical and magical thinking as part of countless possible scripts from which we can choose, as long as they motivate us to learn and to fulfill our dreams. Friendly thinking relinquishes precise knowledge of "truth" and "falsehood" – it is creative.

Let us examine for a minute the goings-on between a boy and his parents who for the umpteenth time badger him to finish his homework. This ineffectual repetition does not benefit the parents, and certainly not the son. Most often, it is damaging. And yet they continue. Friendly thinking, on the other hand, challenges us to come up with dozens of ideas. These ideas focus on what we can do to change the situation and what course of conduct we should choose. Good suggestions may be included among these ideas: for example, asking the boy to quit school and get a job. In response the boy may discover that he actually prefers staying in school, understanding that he must make an effort in order to do that. Alternatively, parents may focus on a hobby which the boy is keen on, assist him in developing it to the fullest of his ability and accept that he may not do his homework for other subjects. Sometimes the new idea brings change, sometimes it does not. However, there is no doubt that the chance of success is increased much more by friendly thinking than by repeatedly demanding the completion of homework, which may be rational but is also ineffectual.

When I tell a client: "Perhaps, instead of complaining, you should get up and do something," I cannot promise that whatever he does will bring about the hoped-for result. But I make clear that spending time complaining will certainly not bring about any change in him or in the world, whereas considering his options might do. And if he tries something that fails to lead him to a friendly place, he can easily change direction and try something else. Thanks to friendly thinking, he stops running in place and repeating the ineffectual for the umpteenth time.

Despite its inviting name, this third type of thinking is not simple for those of us who are the products of magical or logical-analytical thinking. **Friendly thinking demands that we rise above our egocentricity and realize that what we feel is not an absolute truth but merely a way of looking at things, one among many available in the world**. Our feelings mainly demonstrate what is already there within the initial programming of our brains, rather than this or that fact. We might chew the same gum all our lives if we didn't circumvent this ritual in favor of an act of learning, a novel way of looking at something familiar.

Flipping a brain switch

It is almost certain that as long as our old methods of thinking continue to impose stagnation, no change is imminent. The past will repeat itself, getting worse as we age. The stagnation will worsen with the years, like a stubborn untreated disease. The person whose faculties of reference are stuck continues to reinforce the pre-existing, thereby imprisoning himself within his own limits. He will miss the opportunity to improve his abilities and effect change.

It is worth bearing in mind that **when we attempt to change our thought patterns, our goal is not merely a change in function, but one in feeling and experience**. As long as we are not satisfied with our lives and fail to effect a significant identity change, there is almost no meaning to the question of our future. If we have not learned to make the most of what we do and to exploit the resources at our disposal, an artificial and external change won't help. Indeed sometimes it might be harmful. For example, a person used to a difficult and destitute existence suddenly receives a large sum of money. He may repel the wealth in damaging ways, such as gambling it away or breaking up his family. Yet a person who is able to change his extant thinking habits can quickly adjust to his new quality of life, broadening and enhancing his world and the world of those close to him.

It is hard to believe how difficult it sometimes is to coax people to take simple steps that will radically improve their lives: to let go of obsolete thought patterns which have turned their brains into an automatic mechanism that recycles itself according to old and childish programming and to develop the brain into a friendly organ that promotes their happiness. Some people fear that it is a difficult task, perhaps even impossible. In practice, it is not difficult at all. It is flipping a switch, nothing more. There is no need to embark on difficult battles against old habits, just as when we learn a new language we do not need to reject our mother tongue. It is enough to use the newly acquired language as often as possible and the older one will fall behind, and even if not forgotten, it will no longer interfere with our journey.

I, for example, having lived a secular life for decades, still remember prayers by heart. Well, what of it? I do not need to work hard to blot out what is sitting in the storage area of my mind, but only to change my priorities. Identity is like a storeroom which has all our components lined up at the front. It does not include abilities we choose to leave behind. This is hardly a bad thing. The friendly means at our disposal cause us to shed a less relevant or useful ability at any given moment, just as we might exchange an old car for a new one.

First aid: The bypass

One morning I awoke suffering from a terrible toothache. My eyes would not open from the pain, and I was wholly submerged in torment. It was clear to me that I had to make an appointment with the dentist, which I had postponed for quite a while. In the meantime, I was in urgent need of painkillers, which were unfortunately not on hand. I knew I had little time to go to the drugstore, as I was about to meet a client. I would have to ask my client to wait, it seemed.

But that is not what happened. The minute my client crossed the threshold of my office, we started the meeting. Afterwards I had another meeting and continued on until the end of the day. Only towards evening, at the end of my workday, did I remember the agony of the morning. It was the rational knowledge that I had to deal with my tooth, rather than the pain, which made me schedule a dental appointment. In other words, my professional schedule eradicated the pain quite easily. In fact, it turned out to be wonderful first aid.

What I did, without being conscious of it, was a maneuver I call the bypass. It is meant for those of us who are faced with an obstacle which appears to be insurmountable. I see this as an important exercise, as it is the basis for any friendly activity. The obvious implication is the following: instead of paying attention to what you feel, do something you are capable of doing.

Take for example a man who wakes up every morning with a heavy heart. The culture in which he has been raised moves him to want to know the nature of his distress. With a magnifying glass, he looks into the depths of his psyche and rummages around thoroughly trying to discover what he feels exactly, why he feels this way, what is the source of this feeling, what associations it engenders and other equally depressing scenarios. He freely indulges in his moods and deepens his sorrow. After thoroughly wallowing in self-pity, he is a candidate for proper depression which will only motivate him to bury himself in a deep hole. In his heart emerges the possibility of saying goodbye to this sorry life, but since that too requires an effort, he lets it go. If, fortunately, he must go to work, he eventually gets himself out of bed and may feel differently once he is out in the real world. If, however, what awaits him is a day empty of activity, he might well wallow in this stultifying mood for the rest of the day. The more this carries on, the more tired inaction makes him. At night he falls asleep and wakes up the next day with an even heavier heart.

In this scenario, the man patiently waits for his distress to pass of its own accord and only then will he perhaps help himself. Yet there is another way. Recall the aforementioned example in which I utilized the bypass and survived the toothache with work meetings; this man can likewise choose a friendly route, the opposite of the one he picked at first.

So one morning he wakes up with a heavy heart, but this time he does not delve deeper into it. Instead he asks himself: "What can I do to benefit myself?" I stress: the question is not "What do I *feel* like doing?" but "What *can* I do?" Our man then discovers he has many options, even when he is not in a good mood, and he rises and does something, whatever it is matters not, so long as he is active. Let us say he walks the city streets aimlessly for an hour or two. He then has some juice, or coffee, or tea and decides to go to a matinee, the zoo or a museum. These might not make him happy, but relatively speaking he will feel better than he did in the previous scenario.

The meaning of the bypass, then, is not ignoring symptoms but finding a way to circumvent them, so we can focus our attention and efforts on something more worthwhile. No doubt those who occupy themselves with the problems of others, like therapists, will call this move "an escape from one's real problems." How wrong they are! Continuous scrutiny is not handling problems, but merely **passing**

the time. In my opinion, any manner of passing the time, even watching a silly show on TV, is preferable to a constant miserable absorption with one's inner soul.

It is worth noting that to employ the bypass technique we should use familiar skills, rather than seeking out new abilities. When we are not at our best, we should not try something completely new to us. It is better to focus our energy on applying what we are already familiar with. Besides, everybody has a private bypass. If we return to the example of my toothache, reading a book clearly would not have defeated the pain, whereas meeting a client did. What activity would assist you?

Exercise: Bypass at any price

If assaulted by depression, physical pain, frustration or a similar obstacle, let us bypass it. Let us fight for our freedom to shape the use of our free time. Let us compel ourselves to act in opposition to our feelings and *do* something. For that, let us flick through the channels of our abilities and find something which would interest us under different circumstances, or something logic tells us would be beneficial, something better than wallowing. Figured something out? Just get up and do it.

At first, it is hard to overcome depression like this. But with practice, it will become easier. The more we practice this method, the briefer and less frequent our despair will be.

***

The bypass is, as noted, merely first aid. If we are confronted with an event that drags us into an abyss, the bypass allows us to extricate ourselves as quickly as possible. In order to finally get rid of an old wad of gum we've been chewing endlessly, the bypass is not enough. Instead we should exercise the brain, namely, by learning. Learning must become part of our daily routine; in other words, we must live our lives in a culture of learning.

Yet, before we focus on the learning culture, we cannot go on without saying a few words about the culture of treading water, the treadmill culture – one which views the bypass as an escape mechanism rather than as a friendly act.

Chapter 3

Canonical Psychology and the Treadmill Culture

It's a bleak, black world

We are all the product of a medicalized culture. At the beginning we may have a complaint, a problem, a pain. Treatment begins with a series of tests, and then further tests, intended to relieve us of the fear of a variety of diseases. The tests are followed by a diagnosis, after which comes treatment – mostly pills of some sort or surgery.

Psychologists have a similar tradition. Here too the client comes with a complaint: "Something is wrong with my wife," or "with my husband" or "with my child." Sometimes the client phrases the complaint in positive terms: "I am anxious," "I have fears," "I have asthma," or "I have low self-esteem," or "I have a dyslexic boy" or "I have a hyperactive girl." However the problem is presented, what follows diagnosis is treatment – long-term habitual treatment of the patient and his or her various complaints.

In the encounter between the psychologist and the client, many busy themselves with what they are not (not good at mathematics, don't like kids, can't sing in tune) and miss out on what they are (like to read, can cook, enjoy nature). Patients will list countless flaws and failures in themselves or in others but fail to achieve anything by this. Obviously we can all catalog an endless list of what we are not, and still reach no conclusion about our identity. Though some mistakenly assume that such a list is merely a negative strategy of treatment, it isn't a negative strategy – it is no treatment at all.

In my view, an approach that deals with negative traits is wrong in its inception. Even if a person is in a dire state, the therapist should learn what that person can still do, instead of focusing on the negative. Even if the patient's abilities are restricted to the ability to move two fingers, the therapist should help the patient nurture this ability and build a new identity around it. It is possible, as someone already wrote a whole book about blinking. This attitude is much friendlier than confining someone to their limitations and creating the identity of a disabled person.

I dream of the day of cultural change when people will turn to a therapist to facilitate positive developments. "I have come to improve my relationship with my wife," they will say. Perhaps: "I have come to introduce new positions in our love life," "I wish to learn to enjoy my teenaged kids more," "I wish to advance at work," "I would like to become self-employed" or "I would like to learn how to make more money." The goal of the appointment would be to advance and promote a particular ability rather than treat problems, which generally turns into a habitual activity.

Diagnosis and the personality structure

The diagnosis of the traditional psychologist tends to be negative, like the words of the patients. But this is merely one limitation of psychology as it is today. Another problem is the tendency to generalize and define the identity of a person by a single label: "bed-wetter," for example, or "dyslexic." The person sitting across from the psychologist has so many abilities. Yes, the child currently wets the bed and perhaps makes some mistakes in writing, but has so many other qualities. Where do they feature in the final diagnosis?

Our therapeutic culture persuades us to focus our attention on symptoms. The custom of diagnosing according to symptoms has become so fixed that we never question the diagnostic method. Parents, kindergarten teachers, school teachers, psychologists, psychiatrists, doctors – all diagnose. Sadly, the majority of those diagnosed accepts the verdict, identifies with it and submits to it.

Such generalized diagnoses promote the **view that man is a creature incapable of change**. Time and again we hear sayings such as this: "You can't change who you are," "This is who I am," "It's hereditary" and "I'm a type-A personality." Consider the term "personality structure." This psychological concept embeds the idea in our minds that personality is a solid edifice, like a building.

Additionally, the psychological treadmill culture has instilled in us the silly idea that knowing a cause means understanding it. "Ah, it's because of my guilt (or separation anxiety, or this or that complex)!" we say, confident we understand what we need to understand. In practice, even if our causal explanations are well-founded, they contribute nothing to our behavior in the present. It is only through constant learning and experience that we change and develop, despite this or that event in our past. So long as we settle for understanding why we have reached a particular situation but take no action, we will remain stuck. We will spend our days endlessly trudging in place, focusing on the past, not on what we should do next and on what could be different in the future.

Our parents obviously have a decisive influence on molding us. But if we are satisfied with that idea and harp on it, it's like spending twenty years in first grade. In order to continue to grow and develop, we mustn't carry with us only the influences of our parents, which include both positive and negative impacts. We should continuously learn from the people we meet on our way. It is a learning that never ends, that must change the impressions of previous experiences and reduce the relative weight of our parents' imprints. It would be a pity to forfeit the freedom to change our identity and our lives because of educational and psychological ignorance.

Treadmill psychologists accord a special place in the "personality structure" to the subconscious. They see in it the origin of interpretations and understandings. If we are late for a meeting with our psychologist, he will reveal to us that we are subconsciously expressing resistance to his devoted treatment. If we were killed in a car accident, he would tell our loved ones that we had a subconscious death wish. In this way psychologists designate a target after the arrow is fired, and give the arrow's path a meaning it did not have.

There are psychologists who are apparently privy to secrets, who treat the evident as an outer layer that represents mere appearances, whereas they assume that the content of the subconscious is the truth. They "know" that the worried mother actually hates her child, that the little girl who defies her father is driven by an Oedipus complex. It is important for them to examine dreams and rummage through the memories of the past, preferably early memories. They will not let us confuse them with the facts. In contrast, I reckon that the truly important thing is our present: the emotional strengths that are at our disposal, the decisions we make, our actions. All these indicate our identity choices and thus represent us much more faithfully than sensations hidden in our subconscious.

Love, hate, anger, frustration.

One of the discoveries that became clear to me and which stunned me in its simplicity is that emotions are the result of our abilities. This is why the culture that encourages us to talk incessantly about how we feel only makes us set in our ways.

Upon meeting a client, I ask him to tell me how he feels only when he recognizes change – that is, when he feels things **differently** from before. This is indeed exciting, since the person is going through a new experience. Sometimes he is surprised by this unfamiliar feeling, because he had been convinced that nothing could be done. While I listen to him, I think to myself how much all those therapists who spend their time listening to irritating complaints and repetitive descriptions of pain miss out on.

When I was a clinical psychologist, I too would sit across from a patient listening to his feelings. According to conventional thinking, the truly important thing isn't what happens to the man, but what he feels. I was meant to encourage him to express his anger, his frustration, his fears and depression, and think out loud about why he feels this way. In the background was the theory that a person who unburdens himself is like an infected person draining pus from an abscess. If he does that, he will free himself from painful feelings and can then move on with his life. I regret to say this does not happen in practice. Any time I was the audience to such venting of frustration and guilt, the patient merely trod water, rummaging further into his past and into himself with no substantive benefit.

Nowadays I see many "therapy-ruined" people. They and other victims of the psychological culture sit on the couch, breathe deeply, and with brave sincerity describe what they fear and how they feel about each matter and topic. It can sound roughly like this:

"I feel a confusing mixture of emotions. Love, and in some place hatred and a lot of anger, and sometimes compassion too. He's a manipulator. I was supposed to give him a lift in my car to his temporary workplace, so that the unemployed guy can work a little. I got him a job and he considers it a favor to me to even notice it. I connected with him, with his rock music, with his football, but he wouldn't come with me to the opera or to galleries. He won't watch movies I like and doesn't read books."

Or:

"On the one hand I feel I'd like to leave him, but on the other hand, I love him. I can't stay quiet about what he did to me, but then I also feel, in some way, guilty for what I did to him."

What can you do with this emotional salad?

Most canonical psychologists will help with the chopping, the seasoning and the dressing, and the result will simply be a bigger salad. In my view – and I will return to this – instead of focusing on emotions, it is best to focus on actions. The language of facts is truer than wallowing in feelings. Even if we do not understand the meaning of our acts of commission or omission, eventually we must learn to treat them as our choice. When the man sitting across from me tells me he would like to do something but is afraid to act on it and sits around his parents' house instead, the fear of acting is less worthy of discussion than its practical ramifications: the fact that he chooses not to do anything that might advance him towards the destination which, he claims, he wants to reach. I expect him to let go of his fear, to start moving himself in the direction of his target and to stop telling himself sob stories.

Is it in fact treatment?

Because the declared goal of psychology is to help people, then to realize this goal, it must give people the tools to treat themselves. Therefore I do not see the man who seeks my help as a patient, but as a client; he is my equal or my superior in his knowledge of certain fields, but less knowledgeable in others. For the purposes of our particular encounter I am equipped with a view that is free of the blinkers of traditional judgment together with extensive experience with people. Consequently, in this particular field, he is my client, and not the opposite. In other fields where he is my superior, I may indeed be his client.

The average psychologist, unlike me, sees a patient and not a client. The word "patient" can harm the identity of anyone who defines himself as such. Few clients are so neglected that one needs to care for them like an infant. My clients do not come to receive treatment, but to train with a guide who can accompany them on their road to change and lighten their way at times. Generally, in order to change, one does not need traditional psychological treatment; rather one must acquire relevant skills. For instance, a person interested in learning to drive does not need treatment to discuss his fear of driving, but driving lessons which will give him the necessary skills.

Only practical learning will change his identity from pedestrian to driver and, of course, change his fear of driving to enjoyment and fulfillment.

The traditional analytical psychologist or therapist will sit across from us wearing a sympathetic and attentive expression. During the lengthy treatment he will let us talk as we wish, mostly in dialogues that move associatively from topic to topic. At times he will intervene a little to get us to talk, especially about things we find hard to talk about. The meetings are conducted calmly, sometimes for many years. This is best said explicitly: when a man makes a living from the misery of others, perhaps it is worth his while that we do not change. The more troubles we have, the wealthier he will get. Ten chronic patients mean a fat and regular paycheck. Lengthening the course of treatment therefore serves the therapist, sometimes to our detriment. We know of many cases where the patient tries to quit after several years of mental health treatment, and the therapist regards this wish as betrayal and does whatever possible to prevent the termination: "Now, at this point, when we have finally reached the root of the problem with your father – now you want to stop!" "You are avoiding dealing with the issue."

This view of things occurred to me early on, when I was still a young psychologist and had a patient who regularly came late for meetings, sometimes hours late. This caused him great harm. At the time, because I had a mortgage to pay and a small family to support, I had trouble coming to the decision that if his tardiness persisted, I would stop seeing him. As a therapist I thought it was the right thing to do, but the financial loss involved made the decision-making rather difficult. Eventually I took another job – teaching psychology one night a week – and arranged with my wife that the income from this job would stay outside the family budget and give me the necessary freedom in my therapeutic practice. This way I could stop seeing a patient when I thought his interests required it, even if that contradicted my own immediate interests.

However, fairness requires one not to lay all the responsibility for ineffectual treatment on therapists. The majority of people who approach a psychologist simply settle for very little. They are satisfied to obtain a listening ear, a shoulder to lean on and a feeling of belonging. The therapist in turn has a hard time giving up such easy income and is also tempted to settle for little. The arrangement of therapeutic appointments is addictive. When I hear about someone who is in therapy for years because he needs a friendly relationship and is paying good money for something he could easily obtain freely from friendship with a neighbor, my heart aches.

Sometimes an emotional entanglement occurs in the relationship between therapist and patient. The therapeutic process gets stuck, just as a romantic relationship can trap a couple into a situation of choking – unable to swallow and digest but unable to dislodge the food. And for this relationship, which brings neither satisfaction nor change, the client – sorry, patient – is required to pay.

If such is the case, people in ongoing therapy who find themselves in such entangled relationships should do something for themselves and escape. Bear in mind that that of the two parties to the encounter, most likely the so-called patient is the one paying the high price.

In my eyes, conventional psychology is just a treadmill. It does not promote change, but on the contrary – in the best-case scenario, it solidifies the status quo. Those who do change during the endless sequence of meetings with the psychologist are those with growth impulses that are strong enough to develop, despite discussions about distant memories and emotional baggage. If we want to change and not just talk about ourselves, this type of culture is not for us. But this is negative talk. I should ask this instead: What type of culture is best for us?

Chapter 4

Doing Things Differently: The Learning Culture

Learning and friendship – Changing without Oedipus

It is possible to change, to recover from depression and to evolve, all without constantly leaning on the past. When I assist a client in his desire to change, I do not focus on his memories and traumas. Instead I do a sort of bypass: I bypass his symptoms – depression, anxiety, guilt and all the rest – and focus all efforts on promoting, for his own benefit, his best ability, which is not necessarily included in the symptomatic area. In the case of a client who suffers from exam anxiety, for instance, I will add to the existing ability – the giving of correct answers only in relaxed conditions – the ability to do so under various constraints. He will have to answer questions quickly or in the presence of an audience. Eventually, the examinee will add to his knowledge the ability to communicate knowledge under stress.

My treatment of stage fright in a person who defines himself as a singer will be similar. This man should add to his singing ability the capacity to entertain people. For this reason he should sing for an informal audience first and slowly increase his ability, practicing in front of people whose presence he finds stressful, until he is an expert. Such is the process when we move from sexual expression through masturbation, in which a person is by himself, to sexual expression which involves another person.

Unlike the treadmill culture, which encourages trudging in place, I see such treading as failure. If someone continues to feel exactly what he felt before, with no change – for example, if he feels tense for the umpteenth time, not when exposed to a new situation, but to one he has experienced many times before – it signifies that authentic learning is not occurring. True learning changes one's feelings and emotions.

My view includes another important factor besides continuous learning, namely friendship. Friendship is the way in which we should maintain all our human connections, not only that between client and psychologist. It is important that friendship exists between husband and wife, manager and employee, mother and teenage daughter. I define friendship as an ability that can be learned, one that enables enjoying another person's company. Even if our ability to befriend is poor today, in the future we may become experts. Those who haven't bothered to acquire this ability will have difficulty connecting with others. Those who neglect this ability and stop cultivating it will eventually lose the ability to enjoy the company of others. It is recommended that we nurture our friendship ability, but not just to develop friendships and romantic liaisons. Friendship is also the basis of success in partnerships, business and management.

I am convinced that nurturing the ability to make friends from a young age guarantees the survival of the human species. This is because the dangerous and unfriendly tendencies of fundamentalist cultures threaten to destroy life on this earth. I believe that people who grow up in a culture that nurtures their abilities and have a variety of satisfactory modes of expression are open to other cultures. Those lacking such abilities will reject anything foreign. When it comes to a whole culture hostile to another, one which possesses explosives, planes and nuclear weapons, this hostility might become a real danger. For this reason, I believe that friendship is crucial for our survival.

On learning and concentration

True learning occurs when a person successfully adds to his world something unknown and unfamiliar to him, or something that he does not already like. The ability to learn is a mighty instrument. Everyone should keep it in his toolbox and nurture it.

While learning, just as in school, one should do one's homework, namely practicing and taking tangible action. In other words, **action is preferable to talking about action**. And yet, **action alone** is not enough. The important part of learning and bringing about change involves **concentration on action**. If we take reading as an analogy, then holding a book and looking at the words is not reading. We need to focus on what's written and expend effort on understanding it.

Conscious concentration on **action** prevents what I call "repression." In my glossary, unlike the one used by conventional psychology, repression means diversion from the crucial to the trivial. In fact, we should apply the way we see to the way we think. When we focus our eyes on a certain point, the rest of the stimuli are in the background, blurred, and what is behind us is not in our field of vision at all.

If we divert our eyes to a different point, our whole field of vision immediately changes – while our eyes focus on the new point. What we previously looked at now becomes background or disappears completely. That is to say, the act of focusing our eyes on a particular object makes everything else either blur or disappear altogether.

I recommend practicing such focus exercises in other areas. By doing so we acquire the skill to shape our time and our feelings, and, as previously noted, to reduce feelings of dejection and anger to a minimum. These exercises are important, since they improve our ability to focus. Just as we can improve our physical flexibility through practice, so we can improve our mental ability to acquire freedom of thought which will enable us to invest energy in whatever we choose. Examples of such exercises can be found in chapter 4 of the second part of this book.

When we improve our focus, we actually acquire a new ability which we can aim wherever we choose. Knowing how to focus and be aware of our senses opens us up to new aspects of life. If we try to focus on different daily activities, we will learn new things about the object in focus, things that we never noticed, despite or perhaps because of our routine involvement. When you hold a pear, for example, look at it, feel it, smell it. When biting into it, listen to the sounds of chewing particular to that fruit, taste its unique taste, and you will find that actually, until now, you have not really known the pear.

Learning without prejudice

The act of learning is meant to be an arbitrary activity, like fitness exercises. If we want to practice seriously and improve our fitness, we must force ourselves to perform the exercises diligently, even if at a given moment we don't feel like leaving the warm embrace of our armchairs. The same is true of learning, which must not depend on caprice or mood, opinion or prejudice.

Practice matters, because learning is not easy for those unaccustomed to it. If we examine our minds, we will find that we have preconceived notions about almost every topic. Like it or not, every speck in our surroundings prompts a value judgment, for better or for worse. After we activate our preconceptions, these judgmental thoughts are filed and stored in the brain, or let go, dismissed and rejected out of hand. Our mighty brain selects and stores particulars that it considers relevant, performing in advance selective sense perception. Immediately after that, the brain organizes this information, filing it in a suitable section that matches one's prior thoughts and judgments and adds it in as an appendix.

For this reason it is difficult to experience the world without passing judgment. We should try therefore to defer our judgments to a later stage – a stage when we have already looked around, tasted and experienced something similar, and perhaps acquired a basis for comparison. Let us put aside that immediate reaction which first pops into our heads and instead concentrate on the other– what isn't "us" but is outside of us. As a psychologist, I will ask a confirmed bachelor out on a date to focus on the girl in front of him. Afterwards, I won't ask him how he is or how he felt, as most psychologists do, but – "How's the girl? What do you know about her now?"

With a certain exaggeration I would say that if someone knows how he is doing while meeting a new person, he has met no one. This is because, as previously noted, in a clear and focused act of learning, such as occurs in a successful encounter with another person or subject, we simply forget ourselves and are submerged in the "other."

At first, focusing on another is quite difficult. A person who is not accustomed to focusing will find that the quality of his attention changes. Many exercises are needed to sharpen this ability to pay attention, to bypass ourselves and focus on something else, something outside of us. With practice, our ability to see what's around us improves, and we are able both to focus on the other, and be aware of what is happening inside ourselves. We learn to distribute our energies, investing them both in ourselves and in other people. The view will be more colorful and much broader.

Opportunities for growth

Life may not offer an equal starting point to all, but even those who are relatively disadvantaged can advance and improve their lives if they take advantage of the right opportunity. Unfortunately, many miss the opportunities along the way because they simply do not see them. It is important to learn to identify an opportunity. Even a negative occurrence can provide a new opportunity. If, for example, one's partner has left, one should spend as little energy as possible on regret. Perhaps this abandonment will create an opportunity for something else, something better.

Under normal circumstances, we have more opportunities available to us than we can use. Therefore we must learn to identity the range of opportunities, sort through them all and select a few according to our abilities. The world has more partners than we can ever love, more books than we can ever read, more sites than we can ever tour. We must reach a state which I call "rich man's woes" – one where we can choose not between good and bad, but between one good and another good, or **between good and better**.

A person who is used to feeling deprived, distressed and insulted will not be saved by having good heaped upon him. He can always choose to relate to what is lacking and fail to benefit from the good which has fallen in his lot. What is more, he might reject this new abundance, thereby preserving the narrow world to which he is accustomed. An example of this is a man accustomed to feeling unloved, lonely and alienated, who repeatedly rejects opportunities for intimacy. Even if a woman suddenly falls in love with him and is willing to follow him to the ends of the earth, this man quickly finds ways to forgo his good fortune before a burst of light threatens to illuminate the dark and secluded cave where he has barricaded himself.

People like this are repeatedly exposed to golden opportunities of growth and progress but continually lose them. They will continue to miss opportunities throughout their lives if they don't learn to change. After all, learning means adding abilities to existing ones and broadening one's identity. Conversely, in rejecting opportunities someone shows that his ability is limited – enabling him to carry the burden of a particular weight and no more. His emotional budget is limited and he cannot deviate from it. This is why when he is exposed to an opportunity larger than himself, he rejects it ineptly. In this way he wipes out, destroys and ruins whatever good he has received. If he has a moment of fun, he will succeed in balancing it with an hour of suffering.

The opportunity to change one's life may unsettle the learner too, but being a learner, he believes in his powers. As a result, he enlists all his mental resources to accomplish the first steps of change successfully. He soon absorbs the new addition to his life, which becomes part of his new identity.

The opportunity I refer to may be an event that is presumed to be difficult, such as the abovementioned departure of a girlfriend. Yet even a happy event can cause great upheaval in one's life. When, for instance, someone wins a considerable sum of money which ensures his future he has to practice a new role – living as a wealthy man. In such a situation I recommend an accelerated course in "wealth." He must learn to spend money on what he previously considered luxury. Some will find it difficult to spend money on fine food, others will not dare pay for the most expensive seats to hear their favorite artists in concert, while others refrain from buying expensive clothing. They may find it easier to spend money on what they consider essential or necessary, such as medical care, furniture or home appliances. A suitable learning activity for them would be to increase their spending precisely in those areas which make them feel uncomfortable – until that hurdle is overcome, and they allow themselves to enjoy their new ability. Indeed, it turns out that we can even get used to good things.

At times when I encounter a person whose learning abilities are not particularly developed, I try to persuade him at least to overcome his out-of-hand rejections — in other words, to allow himself some pure "good' without the gross "bad' that covers the good and conceals it. If such a man becomes rich, for example, I would suggest that he save a large chunk of the money and thereby diffuse the abundance that has fallen into his lap, thus weakening his urge to destroy the good. I would remind him of that old adage, saving money for a rainy day. Another opportunity available to him is to donate money to a worthy cause. Nevertheless, I would suggest that he do this to a limited extent and not deprive himself completely right now, either for an unknown future benefit or for the sake of another person.

Similarly, I will often recommend that a single person who has started a relationship with many good aspects move in with his or her partner. The change may be considerable, but if they are learners, it will enable them to learn to enjoy intimacy more quickly, to become accustomed to the presence of another, and become a part of a real couple, not merely a trial one. Actually, they will learn to make a faster identity change.

We have become accustomed to thinking that life is no picnic, and that there's no other choice but to settle for a little good with a lot of bad. This is another thinking habit that should be altered. The lives of people who live in the learning culture may not be a picnic, but they will certainly be much more entertaining and satisfying than the lives of those who are on the treadmill.

Say black, do white

Most people, without noticing, say one thing and do another, or in a single breath utter sentences that are irreconcilable. A chronically unemployed person might say, for instance: "Without a job, I feel my life is a waste." But: "I have a hard time looking for a job. I have no self-confidence. This job bores me."

That is to say, he wants a job only if it lands in his lap without his having to take the tiniest step.

We can all find in the back of our mind a mixture of wishes, feelings, emotions and thoughts of all types. In this jumble, we also find a will to work and a lack of desire to make an effort, a fear of failure alongside an urge to succeed, and other such fragments. A certain tension will always exist between conflicting wants and goals.

And yet, we are supposed to make a decision – how, if at all, will we get involved? This is a choice which we absolutely cannot avoid, since even the decision not to make a choice is a choice.

An example of such a dilemma is the need to choose between a satisfying job that challenges us but provides little income and a less interesting but more lucrative one. If we decide, however, that money is the important factor, we should continue to grow in that direction. Thus, we will pick a lucrative job but not stop there. We will continue to grow and then get a more profitable job. In short, if we were not lucky enough to inherit lots of money, we have the power to make it on our own. It is not more complicated than other goals. Learning how to make money is like learning how to paint. And certainly it is good to learn both. If we decide to choose the first option and settle for a lower income while enjoying the professional challenge of the job, we can pick that job but not stop there. While working, we can continue to develop, through studying or training perhaps, until the situation allows us to move to a job that fascinates us even more, despite the low pay. And whatever our original choice, if we continue to advance and learn after making that choice, we may end up in a job that is both interesting and profitable.

But in no way can we realize our decisions if we fail to act on them. For example, we believe we want to make money but meanwhile do everything possible to sabotage this goal. Or alternatively, we are convinced we want to advance our academic career but drag out our studies over years and years. If we act this way, we are clearly not friends with ourselves or friends with our surroundings. We are stuck because the energies we employ neutralize us. It is a recipe for suffering and exhaustion and nothing else. We should define our goals, set priorities and act to attain our ambitions, but not expect complete peace of mind.

Similar to the professional example, we hear contradictory statements from the confirmed bachelor: "I really want get married!" but: "I'm busy during the week with work and I don't drive on Saturdays – I pray and keep the Sabbath." And so he has no time to take part in events which include some social interaction with women. I will say to this bachelor: "You can lead a monastic life and be happy with your life and even befriend other monks like yourself, but it is best to pick the other alternative. Put your whole weight on the other side of the scales and make a decision. You can make a change in your life by adding events to your day where you can meet women, and with time you may achieve your goal. Indeed, you can learn to befriend a woman until you become close and maybe even form a couple."

Therefore, many times we are convinced that we've decided on something, while in practice we have decided on something else of which we are unaware. In the treadmill culture, if the psychologist lets us ramble on about emotions instead of focusing on actions, he will be behaving in a non-friendly manner and strengthen our inaction. If what we do in reality does not synchronize with what we claim we want to do, it means we have made a decision that contradicts our explicit goals. There is a chance that if we understand that, we will rush to change direction.

Increasing our fitness

Ability, which is our emotional budget, is therefore very important for producing change. The process of reshaping one's identity demands an increase in our abilities. There is no way we can have a static range of abilities and widen our world at the same time. Those who are not aware of this make decisions that narrow their world down to the limits of their abilities: when they work, they do not learn. While they are studying, they lose the ability to develop a relationship at the same time. When they bring a baby into the world, they abandon their sex life. And so on in every area of life.

In order to have "both," we must increase our capacity so that it can hold more components that will join together to create a complete identity. Naturally at the beginning, adding a component to existing ones will require an effort, since we are burdening ourselves with more than we think ourselves capable of.

To increase our emotional fitness, I recommend a cultural change. The best way to widen our world is by learning something new, like bridge, dancing, hiking, playing an instrument or studying exotic cultures.

We must not settle for acquiring the ability to do something – we must continue until we learn to **enjoy** our new ability. Additionally, we should learn to connect the new addition to other important elements of our identity. I emphasize the idea of the addition because that is what increases our fitness and our emotional range. To truly advance, we should expand in different directions at the same time. A person who succeeds in combining work and study, for instance, widens his world much more than one who focuses solely on school. Whoever finds a partner and has children adds layers to his life.

The freedom and the ability to choose

It is important to remember that freedom of choice is given solely to the capable. The person who has acquired higher education, for example, is capable of being a high school teacher, but if he wishes, he could be a university researcher instead. If he teaches teens, it is because he chooses to do so. A person with less education would perhaps become a schoolteacher even if he could do other things, but at the moment he does not have the freedom to choose, so he remains within his limits and nothing more.

Hence, adding an ability gives us new perspectives and new options, which is its true significance. Most people will say that they chose their career path of their own free will, but this is trickery of the mind. Common trickery, to be sure, but trickery nonetheless. I maintain that the more capabilities we have, the freer our choices will be.

For that purpose we have to set our priorities anew. We will choose them according to the strength of our motivation, according to how they will benefit us and our loved ones, and according to our insurmountable limitations – which we all have. We cannot change our height in order to become basketball players, for example. There is always a limit to the extent of our identity and its capacity. Yet it is important that we distinguish between limits that are really reflective of our abilities, and limits that were created by our minds alone.

After our priorities are set, we should sharpen the tools that will enable us to reach our friendly goals. We will learn how to decide and choose, always while considering the range of our abilities and the opportunities before us. This is the closest we can get to free choice. In our society, freedom of choice is not taken for granted. Most people have to fight for this right. We do not acquire it naturally through mainstream educational processes. Sometimes it may seem to us that we are free to choose, whereas in fact we are not.

Exercise: What will we learn?

To choose what to focus on, we will compile a list of our abilities. We will ask ourselves some important questions. For instance: "What interests me?" or "What do I think it's worthwhile making an effort for?" Under every question, we will write a number of activities and hobbies.

After we've written down as many friendly suggestions as we can, we will begin appraising them bit by bit according to their profitability and practicability. The more we narrow down our list of priorities, the harder the choice, but that is the true significance of choosing between good and even better.

We will introduce the goals at the top of the list into our daily lives so that they merge with our other activities. We will devote a few months to them, after which we will return to the negotiating table and ask ourselves if the choice we made is indeed a friendly one or perhaps some adjustments and improvements are needed.

With each appraisal, our identity will become stronger.

Inability? Or an island of ability?

We have many abilities, it's true, but let's be honest: there are many things we cannot do. That's the way it is. The world is great and extensive, and each of us is merely a gnat's sneeze in comparison with everything else. Clearly the extent of our ignorance and limitations far surpasses our abilities. This is an objective mathematical given; it is reality. And yet, we need not see the world from this perspective. If we did, in fact, we would despair.

Instead of focusing on our inabilities, we will concentrate on our abilities, which can be broadened, so that we can widen our identity and fashion it by choice. This too is a type of bypass: sidestepping the routine system – with all the thoughts, feelings and symptoms that rise up throughout the process of change – and focusing on what matters to us. As members of the learning culture, we will emphasize our ability to grow and develop: another musical chord, an improved backstroke, new vocabulary words. We will see improvement from lesson to lesson.

It is appropriate to mention here that this type of thinking is also a useful method to change chronic habits and addictions. In many areas we invest a great deal of effort trying to quit bad habits, to no avail. I suggest we do not waste our energy on trying to quit, but on advancing our abilities in other areas.

An example of a chronic habit is overeating. Most diets are doomed to fail. When we are presented with a wealth of food products and we deprive and restrain ourselves, eventually we crack and quit the diet. The friendly thinking method, however, begins by fashioning a cultural change. I view the person who treats his body in an unfriendly manner as similar to someone who fails to shower. My assumption about the person who fails to make the most of his abilities is that he lacks satisfying activities, so he is drawn towards negative activities, eating being one of them. Alternatively, a person who is fascinated by something in a way that involves his whole being will almost regret the need to waste time on eating. He will eat less without having to control himself. The smallest changes that occur as a result will change his identity, among other things as a result of his trimmer body. At a reunion, his former friends will be surprised to find that the overweight boy has turned into a fit well-built man.

Only the combination of changed eating habits and an identity change will produce long-term results. This is verified by Sue's story. Sue was markedly overweight. She chose to reduce her weight not by a lifestyle change but through gastric surgery. The surgery brought no change in Sue's identity, and she remained a person who ate for reasons other than to satisfy hunger. The need to eat remained a part of her, and she overcame the obstacle posed by the surgery by eating starchy cereals and drinking high-calorie juices. A year after the surgery, she weighed more than she did beforehand.

Unlike Sue, Nancy, who was also overweight, chose a different route. She filled her life with daily physical activity. She improved her relationship with her husband and children, took part in new activities with her family and also chose some hobbies for herself. At the same time, she changed her eating habits. She did not opt for a restrictive diet but for varied and tasty food choices in reasonable portions. After many months of dieting, superfluous skin concealed a fit athletic body. Only then did she choose cosmetic surgery, and she is now a beautiful woman. The identity change helped her succeed in dieting and in keeping her weight down afterwards. This success helped her continue to form her new identity.

Crossroads of change: which scenery will we choose?

When we wish to make a decision, we face many choices. The point where these choices intersect is our point of departure, which I call a "learning intersection." Around this intersection, as befits any self-respecting path, is the "view" or "scenery." This includes everything that is within the power of our abilities, along with the range of opportunities ahead of us. In other words, what we can do, what we know how to do, and how much of that is possible for us in the near future.

As in any journey, when we reach a crossroads, it is best to look around at the view, to identify which parts of it are relevant to us before deciding where to go next. We are like a mountain climber who examines the mountains ahead and selects a summit he aspires to reach and is capable of reaching. Similarly, when we identify a preferred objective in our scenery, we may move towards it after equipping ourselves adequately.

The person whose thinking is fixed on predetermined definitions and verdicts overlooks what is available in the surrounding scenery. Thus he does not move forward, but in circles. His moves are predictable. In encountering some unexpected stimuli, he usually hastens to choose something which opposes the stimuli, which moves him further away from reaching anywhere new. And so, instead of moving forward in a process of growth and creativity, he zigzags or moves in futile circles. In fact, most people act this way. They do not live in the learning culture and fail to notice the unlimited opportunities awaiting them at the crossroads of change. If we wish to belong to the learning culture, we should act in the opposite manner: we should intensify the way we view the scenery, widen our field of vision and familiarize ourselves with as many options as possible. The wider the view – the larger the scope of the choices we can make. As a result we will increase the chances of our making the most appropriate choice.

Here is an example from daily life of the need for a wider view: a father asks his young daughter not to use the swing for a few days since he has planted grass underneath it to cover the bald spot on the lawn. Later guests arrive, and the girl runs off excitedly to show them how well she can swing. In response, her father shouts at her in great anger in front of the guests, shaming her while embarrassing the guests and himself. In this case, the father automatically reacts to a specific act of his daughter's. Were he equipped with a broader, more developed perspective, seeing not only the lawn, but the guests and especially his glowing daughter, he likely would have preferred her joy to some verdure and would not have insulted her in public, wiping the smile off her face. As for the lawn, he could have mentioned it to her quietly later on.

After we carefully examine the roads in front of us, we will choose to attack one of them. Yes, attack. The military terms I choose are not accidental. Change requires a mighty effort for those unaccustomed to it. It places us on a battlefield, trying to defeat the opponent. We are fighting on a front that is solely ours. We are, of course, able to use others, hear their advice or receive their emotional support. But we must not confuse the issue. After we have chosen a path, we are the ones who change, and we are the ones who are at the front. With all the good will in the world, no one can take our place there.

There is another important aspect of change. We reach the crossroads of learning while still laden with the burdens of the past. We are like the snail that carries his house on his back. What does this baggage include? Everything: our mother tongue, our acquired habits, our memory bank and actually everything we are at this moment. I call this the "state" we're in. If this state does not yet include the necessary ability and experience, we are not likely to succeed. But for now, the importance of experience and learning is more important than the goal of success. Just as a couple discovering each other in bed do not grade every sexual experience, we will not indulge in self-criticism. It is important to avoid making remarks such as, "I am so stupid, why didn't I do that." Shifting our attention and energies in a negative direction drains energy reserves, to the detriment of learning and drawing conclusions. Did a particular experience not go well? We can take a break and move on to other experiences until we gain proficiency. Then, and only then, may we anticipate a successful result.

Chapter 5

Yes We Can

Homework

Change is a practical process. To realize it, one must act. I call the operating system of change "homework."

Every once in a while we read about a movie and recall that we wanted to see it or remember that it's been a while since we've seen a close friend – but we do nothing about it. A week passes, then another, and we sometimes recall that we had planned to do something, but for some reason we still do not carry it out. When we had the time and opportunity, the idea simply did not come to mind. It recurs to us when we're busy with other matters.

Sometimes we plan to do something more important than watching a movie, something truly important that influences our whole lives. What we then tell ourselves sounds like this: "I would really like to act on it, but I don't have the time (or money or resources)." Often we include a resolution that after we finish our current activity, we will achieve the aim that we have postponed. Every once in a while, we experience moments of clarity when insights about our lives in particular and life in general occur to us. We decide to make a change first thing tomorrow morning, but the next day, our resolution vanishes. We are sucked into our daily routine once again. Another day goes by, and quickly a week passes.

What is the point then in discussing the complex processes constructed of a series of acts which unite into the fabric of change, if making a date to go to the movies only comes about at a rare moment of grace when both of you are ready and willing and there are no hitches?

Any person who decides to change something must **do** something. I will emphasize again that meeting a psychologist and talking about change are not examples of doing something. The meeting and conversation in and of themselves will not advance the longed-for change. Only practical action is productive, and it is only what happens between appointments that will bring about change. This kind of action is called homework. We all need friendly homework that will help us develop appropriate abilities.

The list of homework that may benefit us is endless, but each of us has a personal list. What may be relevant for one might not concern another. Homework may awaken dormant abilities and develop existing ones (such as riding a bike again). It may help us realize goals and dreams (swimming in the nude) or break restrictive frameworks and habits in which we are stuck and so on.

Exercise: our own private homework

Let us sit somewhere quiet and write down the homework that is right for us. While we do that, we should remain open to all possible ideas.

We will think in many different directions. We will allow ourselves to write down things that we will not permit everyone to read.

Done? Let us rest a while and continue the list, then rest some more and continue with the list again. We will stop writing only after we've reached at least 40 possibilities.

From this list of homework, we will choose two or three tasks that we think we should complete. We will choose those that are in our best interests, rather than those we simply want to fulfill. Likewise, we will select items on the basis of their level of "risk." In my experience, the most daring suggestions produce the most immediate results.

Have you chosen? Then let's get to work!

Private entrepreneurship

After choosing our homework tasks, we must begin to act. To help us make the transition between decision and action – not a simple transition, even when involving minor changes – we use an instrument I call "entrepreneurship." This involves making a decision to do something that seems worthwhile and acting on it.

Let us assume, for example, that we have gained a little too much weight. Instead of wallowing in discontent, we decide to do something – wake up earlier in the morning and start the day with some physical activity: exercising at the gym, walking, running, swimming or something else. In the first few days we will be surprised by the alarm clock, and the day will seem disrupted. After a while we will wake up spontaneously even before the alarm goes off, and a routine will be established.

Another example: let us suppose our days are filled with activities, and it has been a few months since we've had the chance to relax with a book. We decide to change that, pick up a book we've long wanted to read and clear an hour or two for reading. After we finish this book, we will find time for the next book.

Or perhaps it's been a while since we listened to music. We decide to change our habits, and instead of switching on the TV after work we turn on the stereo system, sink into a chair, close our eyes and listen to a CD. We may like the change so much that we will allocate at least one day a week to listen to music while the TV stays off.

Entrepreneurship is not a one-time thing. Rather, it is a continuous series of deeds, preferably long-term, to facilitate forming a habit, even an addiction. It is the only way to add a new ability to our existing ones. If someone knows how to play guitar, it suffices for him to strum a little from time to time to preserve this ability as a part of his identity and as a hobby. (This differs from a professional guitarist who is supposed to play every day for as many hours as possible). Conversely, someone who cannot yet play guitar who takes lessons every few days will not become proficient, not even as a hobbyist, if he decides that he has neither the time nor the will to practice between lessons. The woman who goes to tennis lessons every once in a while is in a similar situation. For three years she has taken lessons, yet she doesn't really play tennis, not even as a hobby, but remains stuck at the beginner's level. To change that, she must practice her tennis or, alternatively, take a few lessons a week, at least at first, even at the expense of other things.

This is friendly learning because it is economical: it is the only way for us to move through the boring and tedious parts of learning quickly and attain pleasure, fun and amusement. Afterwards we can schedule the new component among the other components of our identity in a way that suits us.

To prevent misunderstandings, let us be clear: we are not talking about impossible homework. We should all invest sufficiently in change according to our level of tolerance. For example, if someone is not used to reading books, I would not expect him to burden himself with reading an entire book at once. I would say to him: read as much as you can, according to your current concentration levels, rest, then continue. If you do this homework a few times a day, you'll quickly discover that your concentration has greatly improved. This is true of all learning and practice. Let's say we want to increase our physical fitness to the limit, especially by developing our abdominal muscles. We should begin with the little we are capable of doing at the moment but repeat it a few times a day. In a few days we will reach an optimal level that suits us, and perhaps even surprise ourselves with the ability to do dozens of sit-ups at one go.

That being the case, let's pinpoint something which would benefit us, then persevere in attaining it, until we become enthusiasts: enthusiasts about healthy eating, enthusiasts about daily physical exercise, enthusiasts about playing music and so on. We will soon feel that we cannot avoid these activities, that they are not an effort but a need.

Only in this way can we achieve an identity change. After a person changes from a pedestrian to a driver, for instance, it is unlikely he will relinquish this ability. He can no longer return to his previous identity, and it will be harder for him to manage without a car.

Spontaneity? Not in our school

Entrepreneurship, which allows us to acquire a new ability, program it into our lives and make use of it, is the friendliest method of improving our situation. Nevertheless, most people have difficulty harnessing it to their advantage. The reason: in entrepreneurship, we do not allow ourselves to do only what we like to do only when we like to do it, but we do what we can and what is relevant at the moment. This means that we will not wait until we are in the mood and act only then. If we decide that some activity is advantageous, we do it without hesitation, even if we don't feel like it.

Many of those who decline to learn claim that they are "spontaneous," that they have a principled objection to entrepreneurial activity. In our society, spontaneity is seen as a positive character trait, which single people tellingly cite as one of the traits they seek in a partner. And yet, when those who decline to learn brandish spontaneity as an excuse for inactivity, I find it ridiculous. They do not know that by this inactivity they are sentencing themselves to recycling the meager handful of abilities they possess, either past abilities or some they have acquired by chance.

Entrepreneurship improves the chances of success even in daily, routine activities. If we agree to go to the cinema and buy tickets in advance, we are guaranteed a fun evening, provided the movie is a good one, of course. Obviously we can go to the cinema spontaneously; but in that case, we should not be surprised if there are no good tickets left, or if we have to wait in a long, tedious line and miss the beginning of the film.

Suppose for instance that we spontaneously feel like meeting a friend and ask him to meet us that night. One possibility – no answer; second possibility – we reach him, but right now he is busy and cannot meet us; third possibility – he is waiting for a call from another friend and is hesitant to leave the house. Perhaps he should call the other friend and then get back to us? It is tiring even to write about it. It is even more arduous to live like that, where every little thing becomes a complex logistical campaign in the name of spontaneity. Yet when we plan in advance to meet on a particular day, we improve our chances of success, without additional bother. When we know what is in our daily schedule, we know when we're available, can use our time well and achieve much more.

Planning, therefore, is an efficient activity that frees up energy for many extra things. Those who object to advance planning argue that it limits their freedom to choose. This is a silly claim. We can always change a plan, either because we find a better one, or because some hitch disrupts the original scheme. Advance planning prevents the trickery of denial and helps overcome moodiness.

Spontaneity has another disadvantage: it removes our control over our own lives and leaves much to chance. If we want to determine our own goals, we cannot be slaves to chance.

But after all the arguments against spontaneity, it is important to note that it too has a function in our lives. For example: we rent a DVD and start watching it. If we enjoy it, we will continue watching, but if not, we return the DVD to the store without watching the whole movie. Another example: we have no plans and are lying on the sofa. Suddenly the phone rings, and a friend invites us to go out. Of course we haven't planned this in advance, but why not jump at the opportunity? These two examples present spontaneous decisions, but neither involves the truly important things in life. Spontaneity is best relegated to such marginal issues.

With a little help from our friends

Many times we decide on a particular entrepreneurial activity and resolve to do something, but fail to fulfill that resolution. We have all experienced the moment when the alarm goes off, and we cannot convince ourselves to get out of bed and perform the activity for which we set it. Indeed, a high level of self-discipline is necessary to make friendly decisions, and such self-discipline is not always easy to muster. We all know someone who purchased a year's gym membership and went only once or twice, if at all. What about theater membership? Or foreign-language tapes? A diet that has been abandoned?

As in every field, and here too, abandoning a goal can be evidence of friendly screening. We have learned that there is a disparity between what we aim to do and what we are realistically capable of doing. We realize that we sometimes aim too high and will subsequently stop investing energy in an unnecessary activity. In this case, we resemble the restaurant patron who orders a dish much larger than his stomach can handle. He chooses not to eat the whole thing and leaves some food on his plate.

Yet mostly the gap between planning and execution involves inept rejection of the original intention to initiate change, even a small change. Our whole system attacks the foreign object in order to annihilate it and ensure that everything remains as it was. We need to know that when our personal entrepreneurship is not sufficiently effective, there are a number of ways to overcome the problem.

A highly recommended way to increase our chances of success is by befriending people with a similar interest. Being in a relationship has a great strength that can be used for reaching a goal. If, for instance, both partners decide to change their eating habits by going on a particular diet, they make a friendly deal. As we all know, it is harder to decide to avoid food we crave when our partner is sitting there eating it.

Or, for example, we really want to take dance lessons. Although we decide that this time we will stick with it, our bones ache, and we decide to miss just one session. What happens next is no surprise: after the lesson we miss, comes the next lesson and another, and soon we're out of sync. Yet if one has a partner who takes lessons too, he or she will take charge. Another time, when the partner is exhausted, one's turn will come to grab that partner by the arm and drag him or her along. That's what friends are for, after all.

An entrepreneurial partner gives us a safety valve for times of weakness. When one is temporarily discouraged, a partner will prevent a fall, lending a guiding hand.

Another possibility is hitching a ride with a friend with a similar ability who is already giving full expression to that ability. He provides an incentive: one sees how he employs his skills to the hilt, which spurs one to follow suit. And so, someone who wants to learn how to paint will get the assistance of a painter who allows him to stay in the studio when he creates and agrees to answer questions. A person who wants to improve physical fitness will find a partner who is already hooked on sports and join him when he speed-walks. This is the fastest and most effective learning. We learn from the able and have an instant resource for every question that pops up while learning.

Mentoring ourselves is the other side of the coin, when we are the able ones who provide an incentive to another whose ability is still dormant. If we have a particular ability, we can assist another whose ability is not yet strong. In fact, we don't just help him but ourselves as well, as we strengthen and advance our skills through practice. Mentoring can also be an activity that pays, if we give private lessons, for example.

Unlike mentoring, which provides help to those less able, we can also help those who are more able. We help them by adjoining our abilities to theirs. When a boy watches his younger sister while his parents are hosting friends, he is helping them even though they are capable of doing it themselves.

We can even harness public opinion for our benefit. Society's reaction to the changes we are undergoing may put pressure on us. People may doubt our chances of success. They may laugh at us, show off how much better they are, or on the other hand have high expectations that make us feel we are under a magnifying glass.

We can easily identify the audience whose opinion matters to us, which may not necessarily be a supportive one. However, we can use this audience to polish our skills. If, for instance, we intend to give a lecture on some topic, we will take our first steps in front of a small audience of friends or family. After we overcome the excitement that paralyzes us at first and then subsides as we continue, we will become professionals who can lecture in front of large audiences. If we feel anxiety before an exam we have studied for, we can be helped by a small supportive audience. We can discuss the exam with people whose opinion matters to us, display the knowledge we've acquired and let them ask us questions.

If we do not fear what people say about us, but use public opinion to practice our skills, we can discover that it is a good and serviceable tool to improve learning.

The new ability – always at our service

After we take an intensive course in the new material and learn it quickly and effectively, the ability is then acquired and available to us. From now on we can schedule it in our lives as we wish. This ability will be there in one of the compartments of our mind available for immediate use whenever we wish. A person who has learned how to bowl well, for example, can draw on his ability once in a while, even once every few weeks, and immediately enjoy the game.

Now when we possess the ability, we can perform activities that we previously considered beyond our capabilities. Suddenly we plan our time well and arrive at meetings on time. We can visit friends who live far away because we can now drive at night. We find common ground with our child because we are better acquainted with the latest hits.

When we become aware of our abilities, nurture them and use them, there is almost no limit to our development. Let us assume, for instance, that we know how to make excellent coffee. Usually, we are not in the mood to use this ability, but it exists. When a guest comes to visit, instead of giving him instant coffee, we decide to make him a proper cup of coffee. The next time he comes, or when another visitor comes, we do it again. In no time at all we find our hospitality has improved, and we enjoy it. And so it is for everything.

Now, when we possess a new ability, authentic and established, we can harness it to conquer new territory, or use it to cultivate rocky ground until our identity broadens even further. If, for example, we have acquired at work an ability to treat even the most bothersome client in a courteous way, we can implement that after hours in the context of our family. And vice versa: if at home we always welcome the children with a smile, we can do likewise when greeting people at the office.

Itamar, for example, was successful in his career and in supporting his family financially, but failed to develop an ability to befriend his child. When his wife went overseas for work, he was alone with his young son in the afternoons, without knowing how to entertain him. He felt like a bored babysitter. On the list of skills that he had prepared for me, I found an skill from his distant past which he had neglected for many years – riding a bicycle – and I asked him to revive it. On the Saturday that followed, Itamar and his son went on a cycling trip around their neighborhood. They had three hours of enjoyable entertainment, during which father and son enjoyed each other's company. And so, by using an existing ability, Itamar began to acquire a new ability – spending time with his child.

An acquired ability – a sign of what's to come

Have you acquired a new ability that you're expressing in your daily life? Let us not stop there. Let us continue to maintain our learning corner, where we add more and more new things to our lives so we can continue to develop. We will return to our homework, choose something new and just do it.

When a person is a learner, his broad perspective prevents him from getting stuck in unsatisfactory conclusions. He knows that he can never see every item on the horizon. He will always be in motion, and the view will expand in all its colors and shades depending on his personal perspective. Because a learner knows his limitations, he will not assume that his judgments are absolutely true. Thus, instead of confining himself and his surroundings to a closed pattern of thought, he will engage in stimulating learning activities that enable him to continuously update himself. Every new piece of information changes previous meanings and interpretations while at the same time changing the learner.

Chapter 6

Identity Changes – Navigating the Sea of Opportunities

A repository of abilities

Who am I?

The answer to this question represents our identity. An immediate answer such as "I'm a footballer," "I'm an engineer" or "I'm a teacher" bears witness solely to our occupation, not our qualities. And yet, defining the other as "four-eyes," "disgusting" or a "computer geek" is not a meaningful description since it defines a person with a rigid fixed judgment. Identification should be based on his prominent abilities, and so an immediate answer is preferable to a rigid arbitrary one. Yet, even that never tells us about the contents of the mind of the other. No one can be defined as if he were an inanimate object, even if he were to lose his mind and act as if he were a chair or a plant.

Our identity is a repository of our abilities in a variety of states. Investment in learning changes and shapes it. The fashioning of identity does not depend on motivation. Once one understands that change is beneficial, one can reach an arbitrary decision that will have a successful result. I am referring also to feelings as expressions of ability. Everyone senses and feels what he already knows. The person who does only what he loves to do remains as he is; he does not renew himself and becomes predictable in all his experiences. **Changing one's feelings is the highest point of one's learning ability.** This is the product of investing in learning.

Personal identity is shaped within the limits of our abilities. At first, its boundaries are flexible, but the abundance of possibilities within these limits can sometimes be exhausting. With time, as we acquire more knowledge and skills, the likelihood of choosing to remain within our set boundaries grows, since it is difficult to compete with this accumulation. We can change the profession we specialize in and learn something new, but that is not always advantageous.

Identity enables all of us to navigate the sea of opportunities: a woman with a professional identity and a job she finds satisfying will stop checking the wanted ads in the paper. When a man formulates a relationship identity– finds a girlfriend he loves who loves him too – all other women are marginalized, and he no longer feels the need to search for a partner. Our identity filters out what is irrelevant to us from amidst the sea of stimuli. The more formed our identity, the easier the sifting.

The process of identity formation extends over a lifetime. Those who neglect it should expect accidents along the way. The cost of such mishaps is usually high and includes resolving family crises, rehabilitating one's professional identity after losing a job and so on. That is why we should work on our identity all the time.

When you spend hours each day playing the trumpet, perform in front of an audience or teach children, you are a "trumpeter." If you seldom pick up the trumpet, then you may play the trumpet but you are not a "trumpeter." Likewise, you can play sports without being an "athlete" or write a memoir without being a "writer."

Sometimes, a person deludes himself into believing that his repository has multiple chambers. It may have been years since he took the time to listen to a CD, yet he still calls himself a music lover. Well, doubtless his identity includes a little of this characteristic, certainly more than a person who has never been exposed to music. But really, it is embarrassing to meet someone who calls himself a baker but is unable to knead the dough, let alone produce a cake.

There are also identity elements which we like to think we've always had, because we forget the effort it took to acquire them long ago. Who can remember how hard he worked to improve his walking ability as a toddler?

Friendship with ourselves – changing our identity from our perspective

The shaping of our identity is a process which never ends, and which we can and should control. It is best not to abandon this to chance. If we wait until we feel in the mood and only then begin to invest, we will never shape our identity the way we would like to. Better that we identify our interests as soon as we can and make an arbitrary decision to change. **Identity change**, a deep and thorough emotional change, will occur at the learning peak.

Identity change is very important, even if at first we believe that change is required not because of us, but because of someone in our vicinity. In attempting to instigate any change, it is best to begin with the personal domain, as here it all depends on us. If, for instance, we wish to learn to embroider, the needle and thread will cooperate accordingly. Relationship and environmental changes, on the other hand, do not depend solely on us, but on the extent to which we can influence others to cooperate. The person who has not succeeded in making a change himself will be a poor teacher of change in others. It is easier to add social and relationship skills to a personal foundation. Generally, before we develop expectations that our partner or others around us have to change, we should make sure we are at our best and are doing the best we can.

Adding a new ability to our existing ones is therefore an important condition, even when we wish to modify our relationships with our partners, parents or teenage children. Those of us who already possess a variety of abilities can probably make such an alteration without difficulty. However, those who have neglected themselves and feel a need for transformation may be ill-equipped for it. So, however urgent the relationship change is for them, they will have to make some rapid adjustments within themselves first. Only after that will they be able to confront whatever or whoever requires a change.

The question of which new ability to add is almost insignificant. Any new skill contributes to our self-esteem, builds our self-confidence and broadens our horizons. The few dollars a boy earns at his first job are worth their weight in gold. If you have seen a boy ride a bike without training wheels for the first time, you know what happiness is. This is how anyone who has learned how to dive, read and write, juggle three balls in the air, drive, have sex or comprehend text will feel. The list is endless. We should not hesitate to humble ourselves and learn from those whose abilities are greater than ours. Many tennis world champions began their careers on the court collecting balls for previous champions.

Once we invest in a particular skill, we can overcome other small difficulties without much effort. If we have learned to juggle three balls, obviously we can now hammer in a nail and hang a picture, even if we were worried about doing so before. If we have now learned to ride a bike for the first time, we are surely capable of going onto the dance floor at a friend's wedding without special preparation. A single breakthrough paves the way for many other forms of expression.

When we change our personal identity, we violate a prior equilibrium. Consequently, change will sometimes be accompanied by hostility and criticism from our surroundings. When we fashion our identity anew, we should be mentally prepared for the possibility that the group we previously belonged to will no longer be welcoming. Religious people will not approve of a friend who leaves religion, while nonreligious folk might disapprove of one who is "born again." That is no reason to worry – there will always be people who are attuned to us and to whom we are attuned who will offer us unconditional friendship.

The addition of new abilities has a cumulative effect. After a few times, we will begin to feel good even when we discover that we are missing an aptitude in some needed area. This discovery will no longer undermine our identity. We will no longer doubt ourselves but simply move ahead confidently to acquire that new skill. The knowledge that we can add to what is already there is fertile ground for optimism and self-confidence. These two are important steps on the road to the first change, which is the foundation of all the changes that follow.

The homesteaders, the cowboys and us

We were not asked where and when we wanted to be born and which parents we would have preferred. In this matter, it seems, we needed a little luck. When we were children, we were not able to choose our identity. But now we are adults. In preparing to shape our identity, certain factors decide our fate, many of which are within our control. We can and should be responsible for the direction we take.

There are two principal types of identity formation. One is a type of inheritance. From an early age, a person may know what he will be when he grows up. And indeed, he moves along a clear path, a deep furrow ahead. He has no doubts, qualms or quandaries. His road is clear, and it has no room for change.

Such a man's way of life is reminiscent of homesteaders in the Wild West: he is tied by the bonds of his soul to a particular place and knows every clod of earth there. He knows the colors of each season and is well-acquainted with his neighbors. Not far from him, his long-passed relatives are buried. His children live on the same plot of land and will not be uprooted. He does not feel the need to budge. Traveling to a faraway place is a grave punishment for him. If he does travel, he will feel ill. He will stay put in his lodging, awaiting the moment he can finally return home. And if for some reason he is not able to return to his former abode, it will take a long time before he calls his new place home.

In the past, when society was traditional, women knew even as girls that they were destined for childrearing and housekeeping and had no doubts about identity. Men too knew where they were headed: one to become his father's right hand man in the workshop, another to be a merchant like his uncle, a third to study medicine, engineering, law or religion. Even today, there are many who are loath to ask themselves questions of identity. Has fate been kinder to them than to others? I do not wish to pass judgment.

The second type of identity formation manifests itself in people who are in constant change. They mature and have no idea what they would like to do. Their heads are a complete mess or empty. They try to find themselves but never find the answers. They are like the cowboys of the Wild West; they wander and roam the world. Theirs is a nomadic life, throughout which they avoid questions. After a while, these facts mold their identity. An encounter with a new place quickens their pulse. They are animated and excited and continue to run forward and onward. This type of man will feel bored, tense, trapped and dead if he finds himself in one place for too long. He will continue to live only when he returns to constant movement.

Indeed even the cowboys of the Wild West, when stuck in a town for too long a time, spent their time fighting, shooting and killing. These people smash mirrors to avoid facing their reflections, and then end up with fragments of existence instead of a complete life. By roaming the world, they achieve immediate relief, and the burden is lifted for a short while. Some around them also experience temporary relief, as their presence may burden those who find it hard to witness their difficulties. Every so often, a person who seeks his fortune elsewhere will find it. However, in the majority of cases, endless travel is no solution, but a way to escape reality.

Most of us are neither tough homesteaders nor nomadic cowboys. In some respects, our identities are settled and solid, while in other ways we are still searching and remain unsettled.

Unlike those whose professions are the central or the only component of their identities, some people do not develop professional identities. They may take many courses, try their hands at many occupations and equip themselves with minor abilities in many fields, without specializing in anything. Yet, such a man may specialize in one woman. He is hers completely, heart and soul, and she becomes an inseparable part of his identity. On the other hand, a man whose professional identity is well-developed may scatter himself over many partial encounters. Although he will find a liaison exciting at the start, shortly afterward she will view the developing relationship as oppressive. For him, a wife and children are millstones. If he is married, it is on paper only, or else his marriage is accompanied by doubts as to whether he is in the right place or with the right woman.

Even later in life, when our identity has taken shape, we will still lack complete answers to every question. However, our ability to cope with questions and peacefully search for a possible answer grows with time.

Everyone – the homesteader, the cowboy and all those in between – needs to acquire tools to shape their identity. A person who is not of the learning culture is doomed to run in place, confined to his existing abilities and habits. Conversely, those people who know how to learn will make the required changes. The homesteader who is rooted in place will acquire tools that enable him to be more flexible, whereas the wandering cowboy will learn to appreciate one place over time. He will finally make use of the tools he has acquired, instead of starting from scratch every time, all the while continuing to lead a versatile and unconventional life.

Education and resistance to change

It is time for change. We know it. In fact, the need for change is burning in our bones. Yet we do nothing. What is it that makes change so difficult? Why is it rare? Why is it so hard to replace the steak with carrot salad? Exchange the family car for a sports car? Start wearing a short skirt? The answer consists of a few reasons, a key one being that parents, teachers and society have "succeeded" in educating us. When I speak of education, I am not just speaking of formal education. Even compulsive snacking while watching TV on weekends is a product of the society we grow up in. Whatever we experience is stored up in our brains and becomes our default setting. Part of what is stuck in our system of habits must be changed so that we are not ruled solely by our pasts and can make use of tools that enable change by choice.

This is true for everyone and in every field. But for people who have had an uncompromising education, change is exceptionally complex. On top of the limitations faced by everyone, further restrictions and prohibitions are added. Every deviation from the norm is seen as evil. They are conventional in the bad sense of the word. And they are many. In fact, most of us are so thoroughly conditioned that our freedom to maneuver is decided by the length of the emotional chains that bind us.

We are all exposed all the time to a certain educational and cultural system. If this system has succeeded in educating us, and generally it is successful, then we have been trained for that particular society. The socialization processes we go through has tremendous power. In order to observe this power, let us examine social phenomena considered ordinary in one society but outrageous in others. Consider the Japanese kamikaze pilots who crashed their planes for the

Japanese Emperor, or those who commit suicide in the name of Islam who were promised a part of the afterlife and hasten to shorten this life. Even the story of Hannah and her seven sons, from certain angles, is a terrifying one. Consider how easily people rush to defend the flag, whatever cause it is – the crusaders, the state, or a preacher who takes hundreds of families with him on a suicide mission; how easily Hitler succeeded in dictating world agenda, and how many gave their lives for country and leader. The thought itself is horrifying – rivers of blood flowing in the name of God or country, the two principal bodies that dictate the educational system. This system shapes the identity of the majority of children in the world, sometimes definitively.

"No!" – Inept rejection

If we are suddenly exposed to something new which is not compatible with our ordinary ability and we are unaware of our ability to change, our first reaction will be one of rejection. The aim of this rejection is to restrict the world once more and make it compatible with the abilities we possess.

"No!" is our most common response to any suggestion. What follows are typical excuses: "I don't have the time," "I don't have the money," "I don't feel like it." But is that the case? Rejecters do not distinguish between "I don't have the money to go to the movies with a friend," and "I don't have the money for a cruise around the world in a fancy yacht." Essentially, they do not differentiate between an elephant and a fly and have the same reaction to two completely different things.

One version of this reaction is the decisive declaration, "It is difficult." Difficult? Perhaps to those who declare it to be so, but not necessarily for others. The statement that "Electronics is not an easy subject" sounds like a solid fact. We, as part of the learning culture, will see it otherwise: the level of difficulty in studying electronics depends on the relation between the existing abilities of the speaker and what is available in his open field of opportunities. Thus, those who know that they find electronics difficult because they have not yet mastered it, not because it is exceptionally difficult, also realize that their attitude towards electronics may change in the future. It is clear to them that if they wish to learn and progress, and do it gradually and persevere, what was previously difficult will become less so.

When we realize that we are confusing facts with misplaced generalizations, we should scan our brains and check what other areas we depend on for so-called facts. When we are stuck only because we feel there is no reason to exert ourselves, since it is obvious that a particular goal is unreachable, in practice we are missing out on opportunities for positive change.

There is another kind of inept rejection. When we are in a completely new situation, to which we have not yet adapted ourselves, the newness might make it difficult to notice our abilities. Consider, for instance, the state of a young mother after the birth of her firstborn, who monopolizes large sections of her day. She might think she has no time for herself – for a trip, shopping, a nap or going out with her partner. Only when she gets sick will she suddenly discover that if she so wishes she can place her baby in good hands. She can always find someone to take care of the baby for her, giving her the precious hours she so desperately needs. In extreme cases, young mothers exposed to the intense change of having a first baby, who are worried that they cannot deal with this new situation, may react by sinking into a lengthy depression. They cannot see that they possess numerous abilities. Some of these abilities are not directly related to the baby, who will not enjoy its mother's ability to solve mathematical problems or watch a movie. Some of these abilities, like the ability to hug and sing, are directly related to the baby. Young mothers can escape the situation if they take advantage of their abilities and get the help they need. Gradually, they become accustomed to their identity change and their adaptability improves.

Another common expression of an inept rejection is an overly critical reaction, generally with a very rational excuse. Some people come up with an idea and immediately negate it with a contradictory idea. Instead of presenting the ideas side by side, examining each carefully and reaching a friendly decision – they negate any idea from the outset. Critical people are quick to find fault with everything and then reject everything in their sight. But is there really anything that is flawless? In this way, the critics waste every good opportunity.

All types of denial and rejection mentioned here are accompanied by a variety of symptoms, ranging from bursts of rage to different sensations, fears and anxieties. I do not distinguish a migraine from falling in love. When involvement with one or the other disrupts our ability to concentrate on matters that are more relevant to our lives, the question whether the wall we've placed between us and a proffered opportunity is a headache, heartache or other worry, is insignificant. Canonical psychology runs in place, dealing with analytical questions such as, what is the wall made of, what color is it, and why was it built. I believe that the nature of the wall or the reason why a person chooses to reject in one way, while his friend rejects in another way, is unimportant. Each of us develops the rejections that suit us. Their existence is the main issue.

When we obey the symptom and act accordingly, the symptom becomes a means of rejection; whereas, when we bypass the symptom and reach for whatever is relevant to our life and advances it, our abilities continue to develop, and the symptoms disappear without any great expenditure of energy. If, for example, a woman making love to her partner feels pain during intercourse and in reaction decides to avoid pain by eschewing sex altogether, she is constructing measures of inept rejection. Shunning sex weakens her further. In order to destroy the wall, she must make a change. She might use a lubricant, but in the majority of cases, she and her partner can work it out in other ways. They could begin, for instance, with sex games without penetration, such as caressing or oral contact. Along with relaxation and sexual excitement with a patient partner comes partial penetration using fingers or a vibrator. Following gradual but steadfast progress, the woman will accept and enjoy full penetration, the pain turning to pleasure. This is the learning culture's way to deal with intimacy problems between two people. Alternatively., the therapeutic culture would attempt to have the woman discuss her relationship with her partner, her parents, and the world, and not solve the problem.

Inept rejections fatally disrupt the process of learning. As long as people continue to reject what they are unaccustomed to, they will never change. They are rejecting learning. Inept rejection harms one's identity since it makes people much more limited than need be. It also harms their perception of reality, which is glimpsed through a narrow hatch. They thereby miss out on a complex view with many trails to explore, which is far friendlier than the muddy track on which they find themselves.

In the learning culture, we regard such symptoms as expected side effects during the inception process of change or learning – but only at its inception. They are like calluses on hands unaccustomed to manual labor or the excitement that borders on anxiety we may experience during our first time in front of an audience. Therefore, if we do use the symptoms to delay or trudge along, but continue to learn and experience patiently and gradually – our abilities grow and the symptoms disappear. In their stead comes enjoyment, which starts with the expression of ability.

The fact that we are advised to avoid an immediate refusal does not mean we should accept every opportunity offered. In truth, it is difficult to distinguish between inept denial and friendly free choice. Yet, when a person who yearns for a romantic relationship refuses the suggestion of a social or romantic outing, it is an inept rejection. The rejection itself is more important than the reason for it. In eschewing the date, the person precludes the choosing of one alternative over another. Conversely, if one goes out on a date and meets a few times, ultimately deciding not to do so again, that is a choice.

If we wish to give ourselves the opportunity to bring change into our lives, we must cast aside the thick trappings of education binding our brains, and bypass our formidable mechanism of rejection. To do so, we must agree to be "bad" and practice that. We should do exercises we have never done before until we begin to enjoy a growing flexibility. This freedom of movement contributes to freedom of thought, which in turn contributes to freedom of movement in a loop.

Building on existing foundations

As previously mentioned, every change is accompanied by side effects, which we should bear patiently until we acquire a new ability. Accordingly, the learning culture requires that we continuously build a strong foundation on which we can construct growing levels of identity. Therefore, if we have laid a solid foundation in our 30s, we will be able to move into our 40s without too much difficulty. If we set such a foundation in our 40s, we will pass 50 in better shape than our friends, and so on.

Generally, change does not involve the complete destruction of an existing foundation. On the contrary, it relies on it. One of the friendly principles states that while undergoing a change we should not abandon what we have before acquiring something new. One should not quit a job before finding a better one. One should not divorce before developing new abilities, enabling the building of a better relationship. Or if, for example, the divorce is meant to facilitate starting a relationship with someone new, one shouldn't divorce before deciding whether the new person will be better for us than the current partner. (I admit that in existing frameworks it might be difficult to have the opportunity to make sure or to live with another partner for three months before comparing and choosing.)

Where making use of one's foundation is concerned, previously learned skills can be used effectively in the future, even if we have gone a completely different route. Some of my religious clients, for example, harness their abilities to follow religious rules and obligations to undertake the homework tasks I set them, thereby creating major changes. Even when their goal is to leave the strictly orthodox religious community and assimilate within the wider society, they do not abandon the learning skills acquired in their community of origin but use them in their new lifestyle.

In any event, while we consider what type of friendly change is right for us and what we need to achieve it, we should carefully examine our existing framework and the ways to enhance it. The answers are, of course, individual and may need to be examined afresh when viewing the whole scene. Remember that we are not dealing with a table of pros and cons, but comparing several package deals, each of which has its pros and cons.

When change is big enough to shock – "criminality"

"Criminality"?

Not real criminality, of course – only in a manner of speaking. However, I do not choose this harsh word arbitrarily. Although many changes are built upon existing foundations, in some cases this rule does not apply. Sometimes we have to deal with the destruction of the old before we can create a new identity. The extreme steps we must take in such cases are those I term "criminal."

When a client comes to me needing a drastic change, I must know as soon as possible whether he is truly intent on changing or whether he plans to fool himself, run in place, and settle for long-term therapy, which will only profit my bank account and not him. One way of finding out whether my client is willing to negotiate major changes is by examining the way in which he completes his homework. Change – any change – demands no small amount of work, as we already know. To test how much effort he is willing to make, I will give the client, as soon as possible, some serious homework that, if completed, will help free him from the educational shackles dictating his behavior.

Through intentionally arbitrary homework assignments, which might appear silly at first sight, I ask the client to temporarily become a "criminal" and do what he previously defined as "forbidden" or "crazy," despite its being legal. If he succeeds in doing that, he will acquire a reliable apparatus to help him break through the difficult roadblocks in front of him. Each of us has his own list of acts that make him a "criminal" in his own eyes or in the opinion of his near ones. So, for instance, I would encourage a "little-goody-two-shoes" to get a motorcycle license secretly and pay a surprise visit to her parents while riding it. She should remove her helmet and observe their shocked expressions. For most of us, this would be an acceptable act. For her parents, and perhaps for her too – it is crazy.

When I stopped praying, while undergoing my transformation away from religion, that was a criminal omission for me. Granted, it did not cause the police to come to my door, but it had all the marks of criminality, including the expectations of punishment. Consequently, the first few times I desecrated the Sabbath I kept looking anxiously around me, afraid of lightning striking me, or a family member catching me in the act. Only after a long period of time, my fear of God disappeared; since then, I no longer fear punishment for my sins. Wait a second – I have to knock on wood against the evil eye. just to be on the safe side.

What I call criminality is actually violating our own internal rules. It has nothing to do with breaking the rules of one's country. On the contrary, when we violate such rules, we give the State an opportunity to harm us. Almost all burglars and thieves spend considerable portions of their lives in prison. There are, of course, some successful burglaries, in which the criminals are not caught, but when someone chooses burglary as a career, the probability of getting caught is high. The State, as we all know, is a bully, and one should not push it too much. By the way, blind compliance with the law is not necessarily friendly. There are certain occasions, although rare, when it is better to challenge rather than to obey. At the same time, daring or defying is not necessarily a rebellion. Those who rebel automatically against authority are as predictable and dependent as those who are always obedient. Both types do not use their common sense in a friendly and free manner.

Following is a partial, random list of "criminal," "crazy" and "foolish" suggestions made by some clients of mine. Similar to the other types of homework I assign, the criminal homework is also entirely personal. It is relevant to a certain individual and not at all relevant to another. The following list is not categorized by any criteria.

- Eat meat (written by a zealous vegetarian)
- Hunt an animal, cook and eat it – an ordinary act for hunters and butchers, but a horrible act for others
- Adopt a dog – to hell with my husband
- Resume my voice training sessions
- Walk on the beach and scream at the top of my lungs
- Stop working for a week and travel to Eilat
- Sleep with five different men in one month (Obviously this homework is intended for women who find it difficult to have affairs. Women who constantly have affairs are advised to do the opposite: have a three-month relationship with one man, even if they feel he is not right for them as a spouse).
- Go to work without wearing underwear (men can also do that)
- Leave the baby with a babysitter and go out, not for an essential medical appointment, but just for a walk
- Dye your hair in a strange color and go to work

- Play the harmonica on the street and collect money
- Ride a motorbike at the age of 50
- Go for a night swim in the nude

Task: Our personal criminality

We will prepare a list of rebellious activities, things we believe we are not allowed to do, but.

To do that, we need to conduct a thorough examination and review the activities we have been doing on a daily basis for years. We will list those activities that we do out of a sense of obligation. We will then choose one activity and deliberately contravene it, although at first such behavior seems impossible. Similarly, we will write down a list of activities in which we wish to engage but believe various constraints prevent us from doing. We will then violate one of those prohibitions.

Note that we should not necessarily focus on activities which are perceived as rebelling against our environment. If, for example, we tend to swim against the current, perhaps toeing the line would be our personal criminality.

Lies have short wings

Lies are a unique, common and important type of criminality. I do not refer to aggressive lies – ones that are intended to take advantage of other people's trust and harm them – such as embezzling money from people who trust us, but white lies. Such lies are sometimes told in order to be considerate and not to hurt people. For instance, instead of telling a friend, "I do not feel like wasting my time on you," we say: "I can't come over right now."

A white lie is also legitimate when it is intended to minimize injuries inflicted by a rigid establishment which is indifferent to our needs. For example, instead of taking a vacation from work, which might not be regarded favorably by our employer, we can take sick leave. Sometimes kids are forced to use white lies to protect themselves from their parents' strictness. An adolescent girl might tell her mother she is going to meet a girlfriend, when she is actually going to meet a boy.

It is very important to use our common sense when we are about to lie, to tell only white lies and not to make lying our way of life. The ability to make up a white lie is an acquired skill. If it is not the sort of thing we are used to, we might want to practice it a little, but not when dealing with people whose trust we value greatly. This way, whenever such a lie becomes essential, which will happen sooner or later, we will know how to use it.

Criminality is strong medicine – incorrect usage may be harmful. In practice, I only recommend it to people whom I know personally and work with regularly. This is the only way I can make sure that this essential ability is promoted without any damage being done. As for you, the readers I don't know personally – I suggest you read this chapter, but beware of hasty conclusions. Remember that criminality and rebellion are only needed temporarily to ignite the friendliness ability. Later on, after we find out that we have the ability to deviate from habit, we should consider each act separately. For example, people who are used to eating only kosher food and learn to eat non-kosher food have broadened their outlook. However, if they keep eating only non-kosher food, they will remain as limited as they used to be. The best way is to alternate between eating beef and shrimp. Even if these people return to their old eating habits, they opt to do it, after proving to themselves that they could choose otherwise.

So far, we have focused on identity change in general. It is time to examine closely the main changes in identity at various stages in our lives.

Part 2

Part 2

Chapter 7

Shaping and Changing our Daily Lives

Are you unhappy at your workplace? Single, and looking for a spouse? Or, is it the other way around – you are sick of a relationship and considering terminating it? This part of the book deals with several junctions at which we might find ourselves in need of a change and what those changes might be.

Psychology is a collection of many approaches, theories and numerous suggestions, recommendations and directions. I will not specify them here. I recommend, in short, the friendly approach when dealing with several common issues. I find this approach friendly for a very simple reason – it is efficient and it bypasses the concept of causality which so many people dwell on. I do not have to know what came first and what came second. Instead of focusing on getting to the bottom of everything, we should refer to reality, accept the present as a given and ask the following questions out loud: What can be done? What should be done? And how can we promote the most desirable situation? This is the only way to broaden our horizon, improve our orientation and help us make a friendly choice.

Choosing and Changing our Professional Identity

Towards the end of adolescence, after graduating from high school but before choosing a career, we are faced with numerous identity questions: What should I do? What should I study? Which job should I choose? Where should I live? When should I leave my parents' house? There are many possible answers for each of these questions and not everyone reaches this junction equipped with friendly screening and selection tools.

Many individuals postpone the stage of answering these questions and decide to wander about the world for a while. However, they are forced to pay for their choice. Later on, when they finally return home, it is even more difficult for them to face the questions they tried to avoid, especially when their friends are already at a different stage in their lives – in the midst of their growth processes. Others choose a sort of instant identity hastily and almost without thinking. At a very young age they are tempted to join a system where they find belonging, stability and security without exploring other options or questioning themselves about their true wishes. They give up their identity since they are not exposed to any identity questions and do not take advantage of most of their talents and potential. They make do with their sense of belonging and hibernate as it were for years. This holds true for the professional sphere and for many other aspects of life. A rapid return to religion, for instance, or an impulsive adoption of Far Eastern beliefs might lead to a life of unfulfilled potential.

When we wish to shape our identity in a friendly manner, we do not rush to choose a professional identity, nor do we avoid the need to do so. We create a structure of learning and develop our professional identity diligently. We ask questions relating to work, study and interim occupations. We develop an ability to choose from a range of options, explore the numerous possibilities and try out some of them. We develop a proficiency to add one thing to another. We do not have to know all the answers in advance. We recognize our priorities as we go along and proceed accordingly: we screen the available options until we end up with one that will allow us to use our talents to the utmost. People who check the options thoroughly enjoy their occupations and lead satisfying lives. They shape their identity in accordance with their maximal ability and not according to certain limitations.

Before I settled on my professional identity I looked in so many directions that I became confused. One day I thought how wonderful it would be to become a painter. Another day I saw myself teaching in a classroom. Then I became enthusiastic about working as a doctor. I will not bore you with the remainder of the list. Not a day went by without meeting a professional whose job attracted me. I was dazzled by the abundance of possibilities and had no idea what to do next. Had I known in advance that I would become a psychologist, I would not have wasted my energy studying architecture or Latin. In practice, I tasted from these fields before realizing that psychology was the most suitable choice for me.

Moreover, at first I made a living out of a variety of occupations. I earned more money from designing jewelry than from therapy. But therapy ultimately won out over jewelry making. Designing jewelry occasionally was quite fun, but doing it on a regular basis was indeed profitable but not that interesting. Therapeutic work, on the other hand, fascinated me even when it was less profitable. I do not claim that working as a psychologist is better than working as a jewelry designer, but only that in my case my ability to excel in psychology predominated over all my other abilities. Another person might have preferred jewelry making, and that is perfectly fine.

Thus, I have become a certain type of psychologist. Yet, every day I meet people whose jobs I find interesting and believe I can enjoy. But I am always aware of the fact that I practice a profession I enjoy and in which I have become an expert.

When we are about to choose our professional identity, we should avoid several common mistakes. At the beginning it is better not to ask which profession is suitable for us, but to adapt ourselves to different occupations. By doing so we will acquire a variety of proficiencies, which will enable us to choose and succeed at a later stage. The spoiled ones who claim a certain profession does not suit them resemble singles who remain single forever. I daresay that I was suitable for psychology rather than that psychology suited me. Only when we are capable and proficient in our profession can we afford to become picky and prefer a certain job to another. If we are picky from the start, we will never become experienced. In addition, it is better not to reach a final conclusion after a sole attempt, since such a conclusion would be ridiculous and unreliable. Choosing between two professions makes sense only if we have the initial tools to succeed in both. If we can play an instrument, we can decide whether we wish to devote our lives to music or not. But if we have never studied music, we cannot reach such a conclusion.

Let us think of an analogy for that. Suppose a rifle represents the profession we are considering, and marksmanship represents our studies. If the shooter has learned to shoot well, which means to hold the rifle, aim at the target, regulate his breathing and stop it at exactly the right second, pull the trigger correctly with the finger while the rest of his palm holds the rifle butt – only then can we examine the exact spot where the bullet hit and draw conclusions about the rifle's level of accuracy. If the marksman does not aim well, pulls the trigger aggressively and shifts the rifle away from the target – or if his breathing is uncontrolled – we cannot draw any conclusions about the rifle. Likewise, before we reject a certain field, it would be better to acquire a reasonable degree of proficiency in it.

However, we should not overdo it. People who study for four years and only then decide that the profession they studied for such a long time is not right for them have also made a mistake. When they are finally about to enjoy the fruit of their labors, they quit and move aside. If they have already reached that point, it is better to finish their studies, gain some experience in the profession and only then make a decision. In many cases, people are emotionally vulnerable at this juncture after completing their studies, so they reach an unfriendly decision the minute they confront a difficulty or a crisis. If we insist on moving forward after we have gone such a long way, we may find out that the crisis dissipates and that we are able to enjoy our profession yet again. Even if it does not happen this way, and we decide to pursue another profession, we will know that the decision we have made is reliable and not just a whim. In this case the regrets we feel about wasting our money and time will be less profound.

Throughout our studies, and during the first years we practice our new profession, we build the infrastructure that will enable us to develop a professional ability and expertise. These will gradually become the main part of our identity. In time, we will know what our permanent profession should be and what should be referred to as a secondary occupation or a hobby. It is all about **dosage**, the percentage of time a certain occupation takes. In my case, for example, psychology became more and more prominent and soon defeated guitar playing and other occupations. This is how I became a psychologist who sings and plays from time to time. Someone else might have become a professional guitar player who regards psychology as a hobby.

Many people confuse occupations with professions. Developing a professional identity from its inception until it becomes a central part of our identity takes many years. In some professions the process is lifelong. Doctors who do not constantly update themselves or computer professionals who do not keep on learning might as well retire, because these professions are constantly developing, and the practitioners must be familiar with all new developments. Other professions are less demanding and once you complete your studies – you are a professional.

However, until we reach the stage when our professional identity is well-developed, we must make a living and support our families. We can choose from a long list of occupations in order to do that. A common mistake is to choose a job that takes up most of our time, so that we do not have enough time and energy to invest in our preferred field. Let us examine George's story. He has worked in a telephone company for the last 12 years. This is a temporary job, because he has been studying accountancy and wishes to become a professional in the field. However, he has been studying on and off and remains an eternal student with a low salary who still depends on his parents' financial support. He is 40 years old, single and does not have enough time for anything. He still believes that someday, when he grows up.

For that reason, I recommend that when we are about to choose a temporary source of income, we select an occupation that does not consume all our energy and one which enables us to develop our professional identity. Delivering newspapers, for instance, will enable us to support ourselves by investing two hours early in the morning. A teacher giving private lessons earns more than a secretary.

Do you remember what I wrote in the introduction regarding being cautious in accepting advice we are given? I happen to know people who did not follow this suggestion and nevertheless succeeded. They knew better than to be fixated on their decision regarding their professional identity and asked themselves from time to time whether their occupation really interested them and eventually developed their identity from the field they saw at first as a temporary occupation. Maurice, for example, studied history at university and made a living from cleaning stairwells. The house committee was pleased with his work and soon he was offered work at another apartment building, and then another. At first he asked his wife to help; later he hired more and more workers and bought cars to transport the workers. Eventually he was granted a franchise from the municipality to be responsible for the cleanup of various areas in town. He made so much money that he became an expert in investments and various types of businesses. At the age of 35, he has no financial worries. He still reads books for enrichment, especially history books. Nowadays he is thankful that he did not insist on becoming a history teacher instead of the successful businessman that he became.

Task: Work – Questions to ask ourselves

That's it. We have chosen a profession and found a job. From now on we dedicate many hours a day, many days a week, many months a year to it. A few years go by and it is time to examine ourselves. Are we content or not? Should we make certain changes, and if so, which ones?

It is time to ask ourselves a few questions and write the answers in two lists: one list will include all the pleasant, interesting points related to our work. For instance, we look forward to going to work, our workday passes rapidly, we are interested in the activities we perform at work, we enjoy being there. The other list will include reasons for dissatisfaction. For example, we are annoyed by something or someone most of the time and as a result have difficulty falling asleep at night. We feel hurt or suffer from jealousy because one of our colleagues was promoted while we remained behind. We are constantly worried by our future financial situation and barely manage to smile. Our bosses do not leave us alone – they nag all the time, do not show respect and threaten to fire us, even when they do not say that in so many words.

Let us take a look at the two lists and ask ourselves – which one is more significant to us. If we reach the conclusion that our current job does not suit our needs, we should ask the following questions: how can we make work more entertaining, interesting and fulfilling?

Work – What is it good for?

The first answer most people will come up with is money. Work is a substitute for our ancestors' hunting, and most people go to work in order to put food on their table. But what about enjoyment? Most people see their jobs as a must and seek enjoyment elsewhere.

Many people who suffer at work believe they are doomed to a life of hardships – a life which is gloomy and full of problems. Most of the time, it is not true. As a rule, the reality is not difficult, but the difficult things are those aspects we notice within the reality. Difficulties are **not** the only things that can be found, but the things we **choose** to find within a complex reality which is colorful and diversified. If we reach the conclusion that we are not satisfied with our work, we should remind ourselves that our feelings do not necessarily reflect our workplace. Perhaps our work presents a good opportunity which we do not know how to seize. There are ways to help us decide whether the workplace is 'sick' from our point of view, and if so, how we can 'heal' it.

Work is a central element of our identity, and it is important to focus on it because we invest a great part of our time and energy in it. If we do not feel well at work, it means that this sphere of our life is seriously impaired. If we do not enjoy what we do, it affects us seriously. When we spend most evenings brooding about the things that irritated us at work, without doing anything which is productive or improves our situation, what we are really doing is spoiling our time at home. As in any other area, if we constantly think about our problems, our situation becomes further fixated, and we might even become obsessed with it. Instead of dwelling upon the problems, we must consider how to improve things for us and for our work environment. We must aspire to the best, bearing in mind the environment and the people involved. Obviously, from time to time we will still have bad days and experience some unpleasant constraints but the quantity will be minimal. Dealing with the hardships will not consume most of our precious time.

At certain workplaces, there is a tacit agreement that it's simply not worthwhile to be overly industrious. At such a place we could spend a whole week on work which could be done in an hour. It is particularly prevalent in the public sector, where employees are not rewarded according to their productivity. Soon after we start working at such a place, we learn the language of the organization, adjust to it and take on the identity of a small cog in a large wheel. True, the job provides a sense of security and belonging, and if people are satisfied with that, they are probably somewhat limited, as befits the system. People with higher abilities and aspirations would be better off shaping a different professional identity for themselves.

Sometimes we do not enjoy work because of a minor problem that can be solved fairly easily. Liz, single and 35, is a kindergarten teacher. During the first year of work there is a conflict between her and the parents of a student. Liz insists on a certain solution to the problem which causes the conflict. The parents disagree and make a different suggestion which Liz rejects. Liz believes she has to be assertive and unyielding. Her stormy relationship with the parents makes her feel she has chosen the wrong profession.

I advise Liz to examine the situation from the following point of view: first of all, she is only a beginner, and since she is single and is not a parent herself, it is hard to believe that the parents would consider her an authority who knows better than them what is best for their child. Nevertheless, the initial positive feelings of the parents must also be taken into account. After all, they want their child to enjoy the time in kindergarten. Thus, in my opinion, the kindergarten teacher must not ignore the parents and their positive attitude. I suggest that if she looks into their abilities, she might discover some surprising facts: for example, mothers and fathers who play a musical instrument will probably gladly perform in kindergarten. Moreover, the grandparents and older siblings of the children might also contribute their skills. Cooperating with the parents would benefit her personally, as they are capable people, and she might even learn a few things from them. From this perspective – the parents are not the ones nagging her, but she is the one who brings out the worst in them.

It was difficult for Liz to accept this view. Our sessions did not continue, and whenever I would think of her, I'd feel a little frustrated. I'd feel she is one of those stubborn people who declines to learn.

However, it turned out that I was wrong. When I met her six months later, she told me she was enjoying working with the parents and the children.

Please remember: work can be entertaining, enjoyable and fulfilling. If we do not enjoy our work, it may well be our own fault! Sometimes we derive enjoyment from the fact that we are involved in a creative endeavor. In some cases, the work is monotonous and boring, but we can enjoy the pleasant environment and our congenial colleagues. The ideal situation is when we manage to shape a professional identity which enables us to enjoy the work we do, to earn enough money and to spend time with people whose company we enjoy.

I would like to add a comment intended not for employees, but to those using their services. People complain about failures in large organizations. Unfortunately, most large organizations do suffer from complicated procedures, bureaucracy and bad service since their employees enjoy tenure and fixed salaries which enable them not to make any effort. Nevertheless, even in such organizations, there are some capable people who like to offer good service and help the public. **We should not make contact with the organization, but with reliable people who work there.** We should find capable people within the organization and make friends with them. Capable people are everywhere. If we know how to find them, we will benefit from them and benefit them in turn, since their work will become more effective.

The workplace as a friendly community

In most workplaces there are many workers. In such a case I recommend drawing an outline of the structure and the people holding the various positions: our superiors and subordinates if we are employees working in an office, the customers and suppliers if we run an independent business. Studying our environment is an essential tool for gaining success, regardless of our specific role. As in any other field, it is important that we expand our field of vision and understand it in the workplace as well.

The most significant key to success at the workplace is the ability to make friends, to study the people around us and make the most of our opportunities. At the ideal workplace, the employees are supposed to learn how to **supplement one another** and complement one another. In real life, a lot is being missed. Instead of enjoying one another's abilities, many people focus on other's shortcomings. The key to satisfaction and success is creating a situation in which each one does the things he knows how to do better than all the others. We need not be afraid of unhealthy competition – according to the friendly approach, the more capable people exist, the better.

When I discuss the development of abilities at the workplace I do not refer only to the profession. The workplace is an endless reservoir of opportunities related to meeting other people. Perhaps your colleague's son can help your son with his math homework, or another colleague is pregnant like you, and you can benefit from each other's experience.

What should be done when there are people who insist on not getting along with others at the workplace? In case of partners in a business, it is best to end the partnership. In case of employees who wish to keep their jobs, and who do not get along with a certain colleague, although they have tried to be friendly towards this person, it is best not to confront this person directly. Instead, they should work with other colleagues and minimize contact with that person or try to come up with less friendly but essential solutions as described in the following example:

It is difficult for Ben to get one of his colleagues to cooperate with him. The colleague is subordinate to an executive and does not respond to Ben's requests. Attempts to build a friendly relationship with him have failed time and time again, and Ben does not manage to make the most of this colleague. One of the options Ben has is to turn to the executive and pass the problem on to him. Perhaps such an act will force the executive to make the colleague cooperate. Nevertheless, such an act might arouse hostility amongst other employees and encourage gossip.

Ben might have another option – to try to find other abilities this colleague has which will help him make friends with him. Perhaps Ben has been so focused on his colleague's shortcomings that he missed his positive characteristics – as happened to the kindergarten teacher whose story we discussed earlier, who did not try to make the most of the parents. At the workplace, as in any other place, making friends with people means not focusing on their shortcomings. Mostly, when we notice all the things the other person is **not**, we miss the things he **is**. On the other hand, when we focus on the person's various abilities, we enjoy the things he has to offer, although we are still aware of his limitations.

Nevertheless, it is also important to be aware of the shortcomings of the person we are dealing with, whether he is our colleague or superior. If we are not aware of the things that annoy our boss, we might harm ourselves. Thus, it is better to get to know our boss's abilities as well as his different sensitivities. This is all part of our friendly vista. It is like crossing a busy street. While crossing, we must pay attention to passing vehicles. If we ignore them because we are in a hurry or we are distracted, it will be an unfriendly repression, since we might get hurt or even die. Anyway, awareness of the abilities of people who can affect our status at work is essential. Friendship with them will benefit us, while alienating them will hurt us.

Task: Developing abilities

The workplace enables us to form new channels of ability or to develop existing ones. One way to do so is getting help from colleagues or helping them. In order to further develop a relevant channel of ability, we may ask an experienced colleague to mentor us. Observing this person will encourage us to move forward and succeed. If, for instance, we are novice architects, we might get help from a senior architect who is willing to answer our questions or offer some constructive criticism from time to time. This type of learning is the fastest and most efficient way.

Soon our ability will develop and perhaps someone else, whose ability is still undeveloped, will seek help from us and we will become the mentors. When we have the ability and can assist someone who is currently weaker than us, we are not only helping him, but are helping ourselves too. The person who learns from us benefits from our ability, which we develop further through practice and intelligent questions.

The family as a team

The example I discuss below is of a workplace, a large family business that has ceased to function appropriately. Most of us do not run such businesses, but the ability to work in a team is important to all of us, from telephone operators to CEO's.

In this family business, a plastics workshop, all the workers focused on each other's shortcomings. The father and mother still worked in the business alongside two sons and a daughter. As the business thrived for many years, the family hired several employees. When they came to see me, the business was losing money. There were many failures in the production line, and disappointed customers canceled their orders.

I soon learned that the reason for the failures was the fact that the family members did not function well as a team. They were all angry with each other. The eldest son served as the CEO, the other son was production manager, the daughter was responsible for marketing and sales and the mother was in the accounting department. Meanwhile the father, the former CEO, was trying in vain to mediate between the rivals who almost did not speak to one another. He tried to save some of the old customers who were loyal to him while he was running the business but were now starting to abandon it.

When they sat in front of me I soon grasped the situation. It was not that difficult. The endless quarrels did not stop even inside my office. After I asked each of them some personal questions, I did not ask for permission to speak, because there was no one to ask, but I started to speak quietly. This is a lesson I learned as a young man while standing in front of loud students. I would raise my voice to drown out the noise, which improved my vocal cords but was totally worthless in the classroom. As time went by, I learned that when I spoke quietly to the few students who were listening, the rest would eventually become quiet in order to hear me.

I told the family that if their business had been profitable, I would not have minded their behavior. Their business, their money and the way they chose to pass their time was strictly their affair. This is a pure cultural matter – some people pass their time listening to music, some struggle with philosophical questions, and others like to quarrel and roll in the mud as if they were still in kindergarten. However, I could not understand how they could afford all the in-fighting when their life's work was about to collapse.

Well, sometimes money has a positive effect on people. Where money is concerned, everybody is more willing to make an effort compared to other causes. The family members became quiet and seemed a little embarrassed and ashamed. I started thinking that maybe there was still hope. All the family members were then asked to write a paragraph about themselves and about the other members of the family to make them accustomed to identifying their exceptional abilities and their relatives' abilities. A group game in which they summed up everybody's abilities for the sake of a common goal was the only way to bypass the in-fighting and rivalry. Holding the written pages, we started to make a list of friendly ideas and then practiced team meetings in which they notified everybody about their personal agendas and learned about the agendas of the rest. In these meetings, the family members made sure they did not neglect important issues, and the level of coordination gradually increased.

A month later, they were asked to write descriptions of the roles each person thought he might do well, and a description of the roles that they thought were suitable for the others. Each person submitted his or her proposal privately. I was afraid that if they all came together, they might start quarreling again and we would be back to square one. The moment I realized their proposals were identical was an exciting turning point floor me. Each person recognized his or her abilities and the abilities of the rest correctly. Now they could divide the roles suitably according to their abilities, for the wellbeing of the business.

The younger brother was nominated CEO due to his computer skills. The older brother started managing the production line because he had a good relationship with the workers. The father's roles were minimized to handling the old customers, and together with his wife he started the process of retirement, which included travelling abroad and pursuing their hobbies. The sister upgraded her sales and marketing roles. In addition, they organized joint activities for their families and improved the employees' morale by creating mutual interests. There were company parties and a volleyball team was established. The team practiced twice a week and competed in the league. Soon, the business was flourishing again.

A manager rather than a jack of all trades; a business owner rather than an enemy

Even if we are employers or senior executives, we might be dissatisfied with our work. A possible reason for that might be misperception of our roles.

John is the head of a department at a big company. He is exhausted since he does everything in addition to management. He works from dawn to dusk and does all the work that is supposed to be done by others. The more he works, the less the others make an effort. In the meantime, he neglects his family. He is downhearted and feels that even at work, where he invests so much effort, he is failing.

He is right. As a manager he is failing, because his role perception is wrong. He is supposed to learn how to manage other people, while in fact he is too involved with their tasks. For example, every morning he hovers over his secretary to make sure she is doing her job appropriately. He is like a parent who wishes his child would stop using diapers, so he regularly walks the child to the toilet thereby preventing the tot from taking control of the process. At the end of the day, he should make sure that the secretary has done her work properly. If she hasn't, he should give her a list of tasks and tell her not to go home before completing them. If the secretary turns out to be inefficient, he should dismiss her and hire a more efficient person.

As managers, we should study our workers. We should look at the human landscape of the workplace. We should try to get into other people's shoes and see the place from their perspective. The friendly manager will get much more out of his workers than a tyrannical one. Managers have a tremendous effect on the atmosphere in the workplace. A friendly atmosphere fosters a sense of commitment amongst the workers, while hostile behavior and harsh authority affect an employee's motivation. Even if the worker does the things he is supposed to do, there will be a loss of good will and a slackening of effort for the sake of the workplace.

Even from the employer's point of view, the main key to success is friendly relationships with their employees during production. If the relationship is hostile, as there is no possibility of watching every little thing at work, the employer will have to deal with frequent failures. The employees will wait for the right moment to sabotage something. In a friendly climate, all workers will contribute to the success of the workplace.

That's it. We are leaving.

The learner studies the workplace and the roles. He is willing to provide the services that he is currently able to provide, and while doing so, he expands his abilities and is able to move upwards. If the pyramid is narrow, and talented workers cannot advance, it is time to consider quitting.

I would like to add that an employee who is able to become self-employed is better off as self-employed. As self-employed individuals, all our energies are focused on our interests and the people who are relevant to us. Our ability to choose our friends at our discretion is more flexible.

As employees, on the other hand, we must be aware of the whole scene around us. We do not select the people next to us. They are imposed upon us. In the past, an employee had reasons to feel more secure in the workplace. I believe that this is not how it works today. If we have reached the conclusion that we really work in an unfriendly place, perform an unfriendly task and are spending time with unfriendly people, we had better not prolong this situation. If our workplace does not constitute an opportunity to reflect our abilities, it is important not to forfeit growth opportunities. We should take what we can from this place, and in the meantime acquire new skills that will help us develop and then move on to a worthier, more interesting and rewarding place.

Work is a very significant part of our lives. It requires a great deal of energy but it is certainly not the only area we need to invest in. As we develop our identity as workers, we also develop our identity in other fields, the most important of which is our family. Throughout the years we have worked to support ourselves; most of us have become spouses, and maybe even parents and grandparents. It is time we focus on these types of changes.

Chapter 8

Changing Our Relationship Ability – From a Single to a Spouse

Waiting for the click

There are many single people in our society. Some have never married, even though they are theoretically old enough to have adolescent children. Others have married but chose to end their marriage for various reasons. There are also older people whose spouses have died, and ever since then they live by themselves, sometimes until their last day.

Many singles find it difficult to include another person in their world. Others have forgotten over the years how to live with another person. Thus they look, in vain, for someone who will match their limitations or expectations. They respond to occurrences only when they feel a certain "click" or when they feel "chemistry." On the first date, they try to pursue a relationship, and even then, most of the time, the following dates only disappoint them.

Many single people do not understand that when two people decide to become a couple, it does not just mean living together, but making an **identity change**. A person who thinks he can continue to be himself, without changing at all, and at the same time become a friend, a husband or a father is wrong. To become a spouse who is also a friend, we must be different from before, since our identity should include an ability to relate to another person. From now on, the other person does not allow us to go back to our previous identity, just as we cannot go back to kindergarten after graduating from high school.

Needless to say, it is not a one-time move, but a process which is meant to last. Once we stop learning how to be a couple, we are stuck, just as would have happened if we had stopped playing the piano. Our ability fades away gradually, and if we wish to restore it, we must start from a lower stage than the one we were at before the break.

If we sleep alone for a long period of time, buy groceries only for ourselves, do exactly what we feel like (flip through our favorite TV channels, pick our noses, leave dirty dishes on the table and spread newspapers around) we may find out, after a while, that when we have company, we feel disturbed and cannot wait for the visitor to leave. If we have company for a whole weekend, we might feel tense and even imagine a button that would make the visitors fly out of our house on an ejector seat or, alternatively, make us fly out. Obviously, this is not a very good starting point for finding a life-partner.

These self-centered reactions usually mean that we have not developed skills enabling us to accept the presence of another person, or that we have lost the relationship-developing ability we once had. They say very little about the visitor in question. So, if we are truly interested in forming a close friendship, we must roll up our sleeves and work on developing our ability from scratch.

What is love?

It is time to deal with love. The word "love" means different things for different people. Still, let us try to "freshen" it so that at least we can understand each other. The question – what is love? – is an important one which we must not neglect. But before we focus on it, I want to stress that in my opinion most people confuse love with falling in love. Falling in love is about dazzling excitement, but the excitement is usually short-term. Soon, it is replaced by a different emotion, which might be love, but not necessarily so. Often it is an emotion followed by an intense negative release, a backlash of pain, jealousy and frustration, and sometimes even desperate acts, or it might be reflected in mutual blackmail and destruction. In such cases, it consumes a great deal of mental energy from both parties at the expense of everything else. In both cases, the pain component is much greater than the enjoyment. If falling in love does not lead to actual love, this means there is no encounter with another person and no recognition of the other. Instead, there is an attempt to enslave the other person, and when the attempt fails — and it is doomed to fail since no person can be the solution to all the needs of another person — the relationship becomes a nightmare.

A relationship which starts with falling in love is a successful one when it becomes actual love. Nevertheless, falling in love is not a preliminary condition. Love can develop from different types of relationships. In order for us to love, a friendly conceptual discipline is required alongside the sensational storm. Thus, we must understand two things: first, that the initial emotions do not guarantee that we have encountered someone with a friendly ability. Secondly, even if we do not feel we have met a friend, it does not necessarily mean that this relationship is not worthwhile. We had better perform the acts of learning, and perhaps they will lead to love. Due to the confusion between love and falling in love, people usually connect love with great happiness, the meaning of life, laughter and joy but also great sorrow, depression, vulnerability, hatred and many other emotions. People believe that there are so many accoutrements to love such as distress, sadness, lack of appetite, overeating, glumness, and jealousy. The plethora of poems testifies to the intensity of love. The expression "broken heart" seems almost essential when it comes to the idea of love. The protection mechanism – "Don't fall in love so you will not get hurt" — is also very common.

So, what is love all about? I will take the risk of trying to define it. **Love means that two people have learned about each other to the extent that they became experts on each other. They use this expertise in order to nurture their friendship.** Lovers complement one another and do not burden their partner. They respond to their spouse's requests and suggestions, but do not ask the other for something unachievable or for which they are unable to give. They acknowledge their spouse's individual identity, realize that they are two different people and do not look for symmetry in the relationship. The relationship of two people who love one another is a combination of two reservoirs of abilities which have formed a totally new mixture. The identity of each spouse has expanded to contain the other. A common identity has been created, a common consciousness. Each of them feels intimacy, closeness, warmth, support and a desire to nurture the other.

On the other hand, falling in love is actually stimulation – a situation in which we are not detached, and our senses are ready to catch sights, sounds, smells and tastes. We look, listen, touch, feel, stroke and are exposed to so many possibilities we cannot contain that we are overwhelmed. We are like thimbles tumbling in Niagara Falls. When we see the other person, hear the voice and sense the softness of the other's hair, our hearts beat faster and we feel we have fallen in love. Falling in love is in fact our response to a flow of stimuli.

If falling in love becomes actual love it means we have formed an identity in this respect. From now on, we have a wide-ranging means of expression to help us navigate the sea of endless stimulations. Although we still perceive all the enticements to turn elsewhere, we do not deviate from the path that we have chosen. When we have the ability to love and enjoy a truly excellent friendship, what need do we have for all those other stimulations? Because we already love and are loved, we are not confused by the abundance of stimuli. We will now continue with the topic of this chapter – the singles scene.

There's no room for two

It is difficult to generalize when it comes to the large population of singles nowadays. Although many singles are able to form a relationship but choose to remain alone for various reasons, I assume that most of them are looking for a suitable spouse, some more actively than others. We might refer to adults who have not started a family unit despite their wish to do so as people who lack ability in this field. They resemble those who have not learned to play an instrument or do not know to write books. But in our present social scene, the identity of people lacking such skills is not impaired, since they are the majority.

But if people have not learned to form a friendship which may develop into a relationship and parenthood, they are considered immature adults. They cannot adjust to the norms of society, and are forced to spend their time with other singles. Singles who wish to make an identity change should try to learn friendship skills. It is extremely difficult to penetrate the private space around those who are used to living alone. Often, there is no room for any other person. It is easier to dream about love and relationships than to engage in reality. Sometimes such people can form partial relationships, which means they will get together with someone only when it is convenient for them. Such a relationship does not allow them to develop the ability to become part of a couple, because a couple's identity requires much more than a weekly date. But when such people are exposed to others intensively, they may suffer various side effects – a feeling of suffocation, a tendency to get irritated and offended, or repulsion. They do not understand that the source of these emotions is not their supposedly unworthy partners, but their own lack of skills. Their partners are only "guilty' of being there.

Like, dislike

Considerable intellectual discipline is needed to understand the following assertion: the question whether, at first sight, we like or dislike a stranger does not tell us anything about that other person. Instead, it tells us a lot about ourselves. Love at first sight and repulsion at first sight come from the recesses of our mind and not from a realistic perception of the other person. We know almost nothing about this person, and our opinion is formed before we become familiar with them.

I am very picky when it comes to choosing my friends, but I do not select them because of "chemistry" or because something "click" but after **considering their abilities and my own abilities.** Only when we learn about other people's abilities in the course of spending time with them do we have a reliable tool which enables us to decide whether we should or should not make room for this person in our lives. If, for instance, you start playing bridge with someone, you may find out during the games that she has fascinating abilities which match your own abilities in other areas, and that you both enjoy learning new things together. You might as well find out the opposite too. But these discoveries will only be made based on time spent together, not on the color of her eyes or the size of her breasts.

A life-partner is not the product of a first date but will be encountered through mutual interactions. Searching for a person who seems right from the very first date is one of several obstacles we face when we try to establish a relationship. Obviously, one should not continue dating for too long a period. We must determine a time limit so as not to get bogged down in a process that is unfriendly to us.

Esther is single, unemployed, 37 years old and still lives with her parents. So far she has had numerous blind dates, but all her relationships with men peter out after a few dates, leaving her frustrated and bitter. She complains: "Men only want sex!"

"Only?" I ask. Why should she focus on the "only" and ruin the small pleasures she might have for the time being? If Esther had a spouse, her refusal would be understandable, but it is not clear in her current situation. Obviously, a well-developed friendship should include many components besides sex, but by rejecting the men who are looking for intercourse, she is missing out on the only thing she might have. In addition, why go on so many useless blind dates if they are unproductive for her? She must "discipline" her way of thinking and not allow her tendency to find fault with the man facing her to dictate her life. Instead, she must put these faults aside and meet the person several times, after which her negative feelings might turn into positive ones. Esther also faces another problem which makes it difficult for her to develop a relationship.

She does not even have the opportunity to invite a man over for a cup of coffee, since she still lives with her parents. In fact, she has become stuck, as if she were repeating the same grade year after year. Consequently, she must shift back to learning mode and experience lasting relationships with several men until she finds someone with whom she can enjoy numerous activities.

Another common obstacle in the process of finding a life-partner is searching for binding rules at the beginning of the relationship. The answer to the question of whether it is right or wrong to have sex on the first date is ambiguous. Sometimes sex on the first date leads to a much closer relationship, while sometimes it makes us feel as though we no longer have anything to look forward to. This feeling is nonsense, of course, but it is commonly found amongst those who know nothing about friendship. A third obstacle that can block the way to a successful relationship is weighing its pros and cons. For this purpose, we carry out psychological, astrological and other types of analysis which only end up with the following: on the one hand he is X, but on the other hand he is Y. Many people think that such analysis is rational, while in fact this way of looking at a relationship harms our friendships with others.

Bob at 29 looks like an awkward, gangly kid. Perhaps this accounts for his lack of success with the opposite sex. So far he has had a few relationships, all of which were brief, difficult and disappointing. He visits prostitutes frequently. At last, he manages, for the first time in his life, to have a longer relationship with someone who makes him feel good. However, when this woman starts talking about getting married, he starts to have second thoughts and wants to end the relationship or make the woman end it. My friendly advice to him was to continue the relationship despite his concerns and even try to work harder at it until all his symptoms of anxiety disappeared.

I told him not to rule out the idea of marriage. If he manages at last to build a pleasant, fulfilling relationship, he should stick to it.

Ricki, on the other hand, a divorced mother, dated a 49-year-old bachelor, but felt he was hurting her. Though he claimed he wanted a wife and children, he kept using condoms, and examined them after use to make sure they were not torn, which meant he was not sincere. In other words, the man was a chronic single with a very limited ability for friendship. Ricki took my advice by investing a few more weeks in the relationship and then making a decision. She discovered that the man was limited not only with regard to his friendship ability, but also where his learning ability was concerned. He did not pay attention to her desire for a relationship, talked only about his feelings and was not really interested in her. A month later Ricki broke up with him and started dating a newly divorced man, who was also a father. This relationship was much simpler and more rewarding.

It is important to remember that even if a particular relationship does not lead to marriage, it can still be beneficial. We gain experience and develop our relationship ability, just as constant physical exercise increases our chances of winning the next game. At the end of the relationship, both partners are in a better position to begin the next relationship. The questions of whether a particular relationship has come to an end and whether we are then ready to move on remain open. There is no fixed number of dates or other formula we can rely on.

Task: A package deal that suits me

Many long-time male and female singles find fault with any potential partner and miss out on the joys they might have found.

When we are about to choose our favorite partner amongst several potential ones, we should **not** prepare an imaginary list of desirable characteristics and mark a plus or minus next to each one. If we do make comparisons, we had better see the candidates as "packages" of stimuli – each one including advantages and disadvantages – and choose the best package. No doubt, the chosen package will include some faults too, and the rejected ones will include some fine qualities, but we must not forget that we are choosing a person, and not a shopping list.

The technology of love

The journey to love is extremely practical and not a matter of coincidence. First and foremost, we must develop a new ability – the ability to love. This ability will give us the freedom to select a partner. A person who has no abilities cannot choose. In order to develop this ability, we must first find a partner.

Suppose you are single and in love, but the person you are in love with is not interested in you. At first, you are not deterred and continue to court her constantly, but there is no doubt – she says no. You should know that if you are in love with someone who is not interested in you, you are in fact rejecting all the other women around you. Therefore, you should look around for an opportunity, approach someone else who is interested in you and start dating her. This advice is also valid for single women in love.

I repeat, I do not recommend being in a relationship which lacks love and interest, but the good feelings we seek are usually found at the end of the trail. When we have not yet acquired the ability to form relationships, we do not feel good around other people. However, we should let our ability develop and remember that even if we do feel good and fall in love, it still does not mean that we will have a successful, friendly relationship.

Imagine that one has chosen a person to focus on, made the initial contact and started dating. In order to make the most of the meetings, they should ask themselves what they can do together. The question is not what they feel like doing, but what they should do. They should look for activities that are potentially enjoyable or beneficial. I also recommend fixing the date and the content of the following meeting during the first meeting and the following ones. By doing so, they do not have to bother making plans on the phone, they will not be disappointed if the other person prefers a different activity, and they will avoid the power games that accompany the question of who calls the other first. The plans are made in advance.

The date is over and each returns home. Don't be lazy, I say to them, write a report about the meeting, since, as I have already explained, the journey to love is composed of practical steps. The report should include three parts. The first one should focus on what happened on the date in the most objective way possible:

"We went to a coffee house, talked about her job, about a book we both read, about trips abroad and about Chinese philosophy. Then we drove around, made out a little and went our separate ways. We plan to meet the day after tomorrow and go to a play."

It is not easy for egocentric people to write a report without expressing their opinions and impressions, but this is an excellent, beneficial exercise.
The second part of the report should focus on the other person and what has been learned. Here one must avoid stating conscious

opinion and try to focus on the information given by the other person during the last meeting:

"He served as an artilleryman in the army, studied psychology at the university and nowadays works in high-tech. He likes music and photography."

This information will not be obtained by interrogation, but casually, through small talk and through questions asked out of interest and curiosity. The information is important since it will be a reliable basis for future meetings. It will help us understand our partner's likes and abilities. It increases the chances that our initiatives will succeed.

Only in the third part is there room to consciously express oneself. Here one should write the lessons learned during the meeting and practical suggestions for the next one, for example:

"I think it is better to book seats in the restaurant in advance. It was nice, but we had to wait 20 minutes for a table."

"I think I talked about my former girlfriend, and my partner was annoyed by that. She tried to conceal it in order not to ruin the date, but it's better to talk about different subjects."

"I don't feel like seeing him for much longer. He is tiresome. Still, I will meet him once or twice more because I may have become a bit rusty since the last time I was in a relationship. Perhaps he isn't that tiring and it's me who is exhausted."

"She always comes hungry which forces me to prepare in advance – buy groceries, learn how to make pasta. It won't do me any harm."

These reports may be a bother, but they are very helpful. We should relate to them as practical training. They will help us realize our friendly interest so we can relate to the topics our partners like and to their capabilities. Between the meetings we should do additional friendly homework. The list is not enough – we should act according to it. You find out that he really likes science fiction? Read some science fiction books so you will have a solid basis to connect with him. People who know how to do this kind of homework will benefit from any relationship, improve themselves and broaden their horizons.

Eileen – A case study

Eileen was a 38-year-old single journalist. She had never had a lasting relationship. She had had many brief relationships, most of which were just flings. She was an attractive woman with many admirers, but she never waited passively for someone to make a pass at her. She used to go to discotheques and night clubs and always found someone she fancied and invited him to dance. Eileen was a good dancer and a very sensual woman: one or two dances, and that's it! She had a partner for the night. By morning the poor guy would be in love with her and wanted to stay in touch, but she had already lost interest in him. If she agreed to meet him again, she immediately started to feel suffocated, hatred and contempt building until she finally dumped the guy. On very rare occasions she did fall in love with someone. Not surprisingly, it happened only when the guy was not particularly interested in her.

She came to see me because she was concerned about her biological clock: she did not want to miss out on becoming a mother. I advised her to seize one of the next opportunities when a man fell in love with her and invest a few months in a relationship with him until she managed to derive some satisfaction and pleasure from the relationship. Based on these positive feelings, even if she left the man, she would be able to move forward with another man and perhaps, in the future, she would even be able to derive some satisfaction from a relationship with a man she liked. I stressed that she must not dilly-dally too long because of her age and must persist until she succeeded.

Eileen rejected the idea of having sex with a man she did not desire. Her reaction was stormy and hostile: "You expect me to lose my individuality?"

I told her that her "individuality' is a concept belonging to the world of singles which leaves no room for another person. "Practice on him," I said. "When you meet him, there's no room for Eileen. Your focus should be on him, and him only. Do it until you feel you are able to accommodate another person beside yourself, a person you know as well as you know yourself."

The last sentence is not practical. It was meant to make her do anything she could to get rid of the egocentricity that characterized her and to notice other people.

Eileen decided to go for it. Soon a man called Dan started courting her enthusiastically. Needless to say, she did not fancy him. "He's ugly," "He isn't rich," "He's studying an impractical profession," "He's too attached to his mother."

Still, Eileen prepared reports on their meetings and met the guy almost on a daily basis. Once she took the evening off, went dancing and had a liberating fling. A few weeks passed and Eileen still could not enjoy Dan's company. She told me she did not love him and that she felt exhausted. However, one cannot claim that the experience was fruitless. She gained some insights: Dan was not a bad guy, but a rather good one.

"I understand that my hostility toward him derives from the fact that I lack friendship skills. He doesn't deserve such hostility."

This was an important distinction. I believed that this understanding would contribute to the process of change Eileen was going through.

On one of their dates they went to a party and there, contrary to my instructions, she totally forgot about him. As in the old days, she danced tirelessly. She was excited by all the guys who lusted after her and flirted with one of them until, all of a sudden, she remembered she had not come to the party by herself. She looked around but could not find Dan. He was so hurt by her behavior that he had just left the party.

This was an unpleasant event, but it made her confront her level of "single-ism" in an unprecedented way. In the following days she tried in vain to appease Dan. He had lost his patience and left her.

Eileen was not too sorry for her loss, but another glimmer of understanding was added to the other recent ones. Now she realized how egocentric she was, and that her emotional configuration left no room for anybody else. In addition, she realized why a person with relationship skills would disqualify her as a friend and a spouse. Such a person would immediately notice her limitations and prefer someone else, and if he did spend some time with her it would only be for the sake of having some fun. She decided to work more seriously to make a change.

Micki, the next man who was attracted to Eileen, and with whom she formed an attachment, subsequently became her life-partner. She faced all the familiar symptoms, but their intensity decreased. This time she realized that a certain emotional change was taking place. Suddenly she appreciated the fact that she could look forward to meeting him at the end of her workday. Moreover, she realized she was getting used to his body, which she had not really liked at first (mostly because she found him too short), and their sex life became more pleasurable. A few months later the two decided to move in together and passed the "admissions boards" of friends and family. Not everybody supported their new relationship, but Eileen and Micki were determined. Our meetings continued every few weeks. She seemed very content. During one of the meetings, overwhelmed by her new ability to change, she told me she loved the guy.

However, she realized the full extent of the change she had made when she went to a party with him. As always, she noticed the signals put out by men, but although they caused some excitement, they did not confuse her. The signals which were once the ultimate excitement for her could not compete with her relationship with Micki, which was the most fulfilling thing. Eileen and Micki got married six months later.

A relationship is formed

When our relationship ability is created, we are the first ones to know. A wonderful feeling tells us that.

Now, the aim is to move on from being friends to becoming experts in one another. When two people meet, each brings along a dowry of abilities which were created before they knew one another. Realizing, as a newly formed couple, how to seize the opportunity, relate to each other's abilities, and use even a small portion of what the other can offer, they may kill two birds with one stone. The horizons of both will be broadened and enriched in a mutually beneficial way. Together they may create a social and cultural infrastructure which will enable them to enjoy each other even more.

In addition, they will learn how to enjoy happy times together in many different ways. Even if one does not spend time on the exact same activity but stays nearby while the other is busy with something else, they will feel pleasantly at ease. Partners who acquire the ability to give one another some space have learned not to burden one another. They do not wear each other out, and this benefits their emotional budget. Obviously, sometimes an unpleasant event such as a bereavement or accident can also draw people closer together.

As I explained earlier, people who lack experience in long intimate companionship cannot create friendships easily. People who are not skilled in intimate relationships sometimes view their partners as burdens. Let us imagine ourselves practicing weightlifting until we become skilled. We should continue the effort, until we no longer consider our spouses' presence onerous but a valuable addition. Remember, the formation of mutual identity is done by connecting several abilities. It is not about making change in a particular area, but rather in a whole system: we do not promote our relationship ability as an isolated factor. Instead, we should continue to revamp and improve other areas of our lives. Remember Esther? The single woman who used to go on many blind dates? She, for example, needed to learn how to love, to move to her own apartment, to find a job, and to start leading a more independent life – and to work on all of these projects simultaneously.

Society's "kosher" stamp

An identity change, from a single to a spouse, requires dealing with not only the difficulties involved in the process but also public opinion. The reaction of the people around us to the change we have undergone may put pressure on us. People might underestimate our chances of success, ridicule us, be patronizing, or express exaggerated expectations which make us feel that our every move is being watched. Parents and married friends may act consciously and unconsciously to put an end to the relationship. They find fault with our partners with the aim of rejecting or eliminating them. Drawing our attention to the things a person lacks and ignoring their good qualities is the easiest way to criticize a person. In fact, these critics simply do not know how to deal with the single who has taken on a new identity.

Often I find myself fighting an endless barrage of nasty, unfounded resistance to change. It seems that as in the popular TV series *Seinfeld*, there is no need to explain: each time a character tries to build a new relationship, so-called friends help him or her **not** to succeed. In the series it is at least amusing. It is far less amusing when a 40-year-old single woman who has become close friends with a divorced man, the father of a child, breaks the good news to her mother. In this case the poor woman only gets the sour-faced comment: "Couldn't you find someone better?"

I listen to the story and think that the mother is a fool who does not love her daughter and cannot share her happiness. The relationship ability of the daughter has only just started to develop – a thin fragile layer above all the numerous causes that prevented her from building a relationship before. It is so easy to ruin it.

Public opinion may also include pressure applied by well-meaning busybodies: "You're next!" "When will it be your turn?" It is well known that such pressure is far from helpful. If at least one of the spouses has children from a former relationship, the children might also apply pressure of their own.

People in the midst of change must take into account the fact that they are disturbing some kind of ecological balance – social and familial – and must learn how to deal with the situation. One option is to replace friends with new ones or select friends who are able to be supportive even after a change of status.

Mary, a 39-year-old in sales, was a single woman who only had partial, short-term relationships and spent long periods on her own. Throughout the years she had tried various psychological therapies, but nothing changed. She came to see me after a year-long relationship during which she lived with a 44-year-old divorced businessman who had two children. At first the two of them had a good time together and enjoyed each other's company. However, when she started talking about her wish to start a family, her partner did not react. Friends who were married women and mothers kept talking about her "biological clock" and pressured her to "talk business" with her spouse. Mary started nagging her partner, until he made it clear that the timing was not right for him. He suggested that they break up so as not to delay her plans further. Three days afterwards Mary moved out and was proud of her rapid reorganization.

While we talked I got the impression that prior to the crisis which led to their break-up, the two had had a good and worthwhile relationship. I asked her why she was in such a hurry to end it.

"I really want kids and feel my time is running out. In two or three years it might be complicated to get pregnant. In four years' time, maybe even impossible."

I told her that to assert that at her age she could not waste any more time was a spurious claim. In fact, she had caused a greater waste of time. How many months would go by before she managed to build another relationship, with another man, and reach the position she had already been in with her last partner? I thought she had given up what she had and gained nothing in return. I further maintained that nowadays there were ways to become a mother without a spouse. Perhaps it would be easier and more fulfilling to raise a child as a single parent than to raise a child with a hastily-chosen spouse. The latter might agree to have a child but be unfriendly as far as Mary was concerned.

I suggested she try renewing her relationship with her former partner, and if she managed to do so, she should enjoy the relationship and try not to complain. Later on she could decide to leave him and become a mother if she still wanted to. And who knows? Perhaps after a while, he would change his mind about having a child with her.

She got back together with him. They had an incomplete relationship that with time became crucial but not as whole as it used to be. As of now, she still does not have children. Most of her friends have accepted her decision, and those who do not approve hear from her only when she calls them before the holidays. Once close friends, they have become mere acquaintances.

Task: Public opinion as an efficient tool

We can enlist communal opinion as a tool to produce friendly goals. Although communal opinion sometimes presents a problem, we can transform it into a tool that will help us succeed. We can easily identify the audience whose opinion is important to us. It will not necessarily be supportive. However, sometimes the same community that makes us nervous might motivate us.

For the sake of a good relationship, it is important to make contact with other people. A relationship where partners avoid presenting each other to an unsympathetic community may fail. Communal opinion can ultimately become a friendly element for the new couple. For example, they can use the reactions of prickly, unsupportive parents to make their relationship stronger. If they keep visiting those parents as a couple, they will get to know the strong elements in their relationship and appreciate the support they give one another. Likewise, if they protect their partners against unsympathetic friends by mentioning their positive traits, they will soon see their qualities more clearly.

In addition, communal opinion may assist in many other ways. If we intend to give a lecture, for instance, we should first rehearse it in front of a small audience of friends or family. After we overcome the excitement which tends to paralyze us at first, we will become pros and be able to give lectures in front of a larger audience.

***

We started as singles and became spouses who know how to enjoy their new relationship. Is this the happy end we were expecting? And from now on, will we live happily ever after?

Chapter 9

Changing the Relationship – Learning to Be Friends

It is not simple to maintain a long-term relationship, especially in a world where social interaction includes numerous temptations and opportunities. Very few couples know how to maintain a friendship that is fascinating and entertaining and characterized by mutual satisfaction and self-expression. Such a relationship allows no competition.

Two experienced learners are able to learn from each other gradually so that each of them will eventually acquire the other's abilities. They constitute a vast reservoir of abilities since they **add** to each other. These reserves are the basis for the excellent, entertaining quality of their partnership. They know how to enjoy each other without bounds and raise their children happily. This is a partnership for life where both partners can cope with challenges and crises successfully.

Both partners become enriched and their relationship shares channels of interest. In certain areas they choose to depend on each other, and they complement each other. They know how to act in the best interests of their partner. They also know how to act in their best interests as a couple, which means their common interests. They do not make do with the resources each of them has, nor with their shared reservoir of resources, but develop further in the most important areas. They add on whatever seems of value to them, from a new position in bed to a cooking course they both attend. They know how to freshen up their life as a couple and maintain progress. Their friendship is rewarding, entertaining and hard to compete with. External stimuli have their appeal, but are non-threatening to the partners. Just as our appetites are stimulated upon smelling the pleasant aroma of cooked food on our way to dinner, so when one partner meets a man or a woman who appears appealing, this is eventually expressed by greater satisfaction in a stable relationship with the significant other.

Task: Mutual learning

Are we trying to lose weight, to learn dancing or to achieve some other goal, and finding it difficult? Let us try to do that together with our partners. When partners act in unison, they are greatly empowered. They significantly increase their chances of meeting their goals and, at the same time, enhance their relationship.

If, for instance, one decides to change eating habits and choose a particular diet, he or she is able to make a friendly deal which will benefit both partners. It is much harder to avoid a certain delicacy when our spouses sit there consuming it in front of our eyes. Moreover, our spouses, as our partners in management, act as our backup in moments of weakness. When we face temporary infirmity, our spouses will prevent our falling, offer us a hand and lead us on to the next phase of learning. In a case where our partners are exhausted, it will be our turn to catch them and steer the way through. As a rule, it is highly recommended that a project be undertaken by two people, since this significantly increases the chances of success. It is also true for projects undertaken by two friends (not necessarily a couple), by a parent and a child or any other couple which shares a particular goal.

Spouses who are not friends

Many of the couples surrounding us are not friends, even if they manage to survive as a stable couple for many years. At first glance, the long duration of their relationship seems to testify to their success as a couple. In practice, the main reason for their lasting relationship is that most couples make do with belonging to one another. They live side by side for years like living-room furniture. In fact, they do fulfill roles in the relationship, but they are not really partners. Each one does his or her own thing according to habit. The emphasis is on performing one's duties and meeting demands rather than on satisfaction and fulfillment. They quote sayings such as "Life is no picnic" and "Life is not a bed of roses."

A partnership like that is in fact a connection between two people who are committed to making do with little . They remain limited within the relationship. When there is no constant nurturing of a relationship, we will find negligence which might lead to "accidents," leading subsequently to a breakup of the relationship. An example of such an "accident" is a romantic involvement of one of the spouses with another person. Those who believe that once a couple gets married, their courtship period ends, are of course mistaken. Couples who do not know how to renew and refresh their relationship are doomed to failure, or at least to a limited relationship.

Here as well, people must not act according to their feelings but according to a friendly outlook. We feel good together and are excited by the presence of the other person? Good. After a while the relationship becomes mediocre and routine. Then we grow slack and lazy. We simply do not want to bother. If this neglect continues, it creates an obstruction which we will later find difficult to overcome. Most couples face crisis situations simply because they forgot to attend to their relationship and cultivate it.

Fights and their meanings

Many couples do not delude themselves – they are aware of the fact that they do not have a good relationship but still continue to live together, day after day. Sometimes they do not fight, since one of them submits completely to the other, or because they are too exhausted to do so. Other couples fight endlessly and devote all their energy to destruction, mutual torpedoing and power struggles.

In my opinion, fights are popular entertainment for people who do not bother to develop a more interesting mutual pastime. I refer not to the content of the fights, but to their high frequency. People who know how to have a good time will not destroy their potential by fighting and arguing. If spouses spend four hours together, have a great time for one hour and devote three hours to fights, it means that the mental budget or allocation they devote to enjoying their partner is only sufficient for one hour. When this scenario becomes routine, the results are an unbearable life and miserable children who are forced to live in such an atmosphere.

The solution consists of two alternatives. Those who reject change will settle for separate paths and a weakening of the relationship.

More cooperative spouses will opt to expand their ability to spend time together, enabling them to enjoy each other's company and reducing their tendency to fight.

Fighting is not merely entertainment. It is also a kind of communication. When quarrelling spouses complain that they do not communicate, it is like an unsuccessful joke. As a matter of fact, they communicate really well. They respond to every word uttered by the other, to their tone of voice and even to the blink of their eye. If, for instance, we do not speak Hungarian, we cannot talk to a person who only speaks Hungarian, nor are we able to quarrel with him. When spouses are fighting, it means they have a common language and that they communicate well with each other.

Often a fight means that at least one of the spouses has exhausted their mental budget for intimate entertainment. If, for instance, after watching a movie, you choose to discuss a future get-together with friends, and your spouse's mental budget for the evening has been exhausted, your proposal might turn into an argument. Both sides will lose. If you had not brought up the get-together, you could have continued to have a good time.

When dynamics between partners are based on a prolonged conflict, I do not see the point of dwelling upon the quarrels, since in fact these fights are like a blog, and each one might have a different version of events. I do not get into who is right and who is wrong. Dealing with their endless complaints will only fixate them further, encouraging them to use the same language they have been using until now.

Traditional therapy is a chronic business that contributes to the therapist's bank account but usually does not help the client.

Instead, it is best to deal with the following question: what should the partners do to extricate themselves from the cycle of quarrels?

Task: Minimizing quarrels

If we often fight but are not in the midst of a prolonged fight 24/7, we have the capacity to reduce the frequency of the quarrels.

To begin with, we should choose an arbitrary management policy which will fill our time with various occupations. This way, our entire schedule will be filled with friendly activities. Preferably, there will be shared occupations, so that each partner can increase their range of abilities and acquire new abilities from the other. If we do not act this way, our shared world will rapidly shrink.

Once we become experts on each other, a new path will open. Whenever we expect an argument, we will deliberately initiate a temporary separation without fights. For instance, the woman will read a book, and the man will go to sleep. There will be no hurt feelings whose expression requires a waste of energy. Later, our meeting will be more fulfilling, and both of us will come equipped with a new mental budget.

The language of complaints

Perhaps the spouses quarrel in English or in Hebrew, or perhaps they quarrel in some other language, but they usually use what I call "the language of complaints." This is the formal lexicon used to accuse others, and it is used everywhere. The number of speakers using this language is even greater than the number of speakers of Chinese. The language of complaints is chosen by two people who agree not to enjoy one another, to look for each other's weaknesses, to attack each other and to defend themselves. These speakers believe that they are interested in improving their lives, and if only someone would listen to their justifiable complaints, their situation would improve. In fact, they are stuck in one place and refuse to progress. People who communicate with one another in this language attract an audience of bystanders, such as psychologists and so-called best friends, to listen to them and to identify with them.

If we examine this language using a broad view or outlook, we will immediately find out that it is, in fact, one of the most lethal rejection tools. Let us take, for example, a person who always arrives late. There is always a counterpart who waits for him, chews his fingernails, and walks around restlessly with his mind full of complaints and increasing hostility that will inevitably result in an outburst. So, when the other person finally arrives, and the partners can start enjoying each other, the complainer turns the **remaining time** into a negative experience. The language of complaints ruins the evening for both spouses. I refuse to cooperate with that. Fortunately, in reality, the objects of all these complaints are not absolute monsters. Sometimes I tell the complainers: "Your partner does all sorts of annoying things, but that's because they are a good friend of yours. They know what you like and now they are just delivering the goods."

Sometimes, however, it is worthwhile for people to listen to the complaints directed at them. People who always arrive late need to change, because in crucial situations no one will wait for them. While the earth continues to revolve around the sun, they might miss significant things. If they are late for a movie or a play, they will miss the beginning. It is difficult to calculate how many things they have missed out on in total. In addition, others perceive them as unreliable and do not trust them. To stop being late all the time, these people must perform a simple learning activity. All they have to do is behave as if their important meetings were scheduled to start one hour earlier. And so, within one day they will become punctual. After a while, this ability will become routine, and people who used to perceive them as latecomers will internalize the change and forget all about their previous identity. They can also become punctual people who arrive late — as most people do — when a delay occurs which is beyond their control.

In general, I recommend that my clients listen to the nature of the complaint and ask themselves whether they can learn something from it. Perhaps they can.

However, the complainers also need to change, sometimes even more urgently than the other side. They suffer from a common delusion. Their field of vision has been limited, and they perceive only one type of information and fail to notice anything else. Whenever I come across a chronic complainer, I ask them a direct question: "Can you say something positive about your wife?" or "Can you say something positive about your husband?" A person whose brain is poisoned will find it difficult to answer such a question.

In general, complainers do not direct their complaints only at one person, even though the person who is closest to them is the most slandered. Usually, they are not pleased with anything. They may at times praise certain people, but these people are usually so remote that the compliments they pay them only serve as points of comparison to the weaknesses of the people with whom they are forced to share their lives. Even when they witness something positive, they will soon become disappointed with it and manage to find fault. They find it difficult to enjoy themselves and tend to irritate people around them. Meanwhile, the partner who expects a negative reaction does not bother to change and ceases to pay attention, even when an important complaint is presented amid all the insignificant ones.

It is important to realize that change is possible. Whenever someone arrives late, we can spend our time pleasantly instead of just waiting and thinking hostile thoughts. We can use the time for reading and so on, and when the other person finally arrives, we can immediately start enjoying our time together. We can also leave a friendly note at home: "Dear, I went out. Don't wait up for me. I'll be home late." Perhaps if the person who is always late finds out that no one is anxiously awaiting him, he will plan his schedule better so as not to miss the meeting with his partner. We can agree to meet at five o'clock to see a movie that starts at seven. This way, even if our partner is late, we will still make it on time. Indeed, this is a friendly change.

Changing one of the partners – "I cannot stand him!"

If we wish to make changes in our relationship, we must start with ourselves. Sitting idly by waiting for our spouse to change will not help. If, for instance, we think there are not enough affectionate acts in our relationship, perhaps we should be the one who brings home a bouquet of flowers once a week.

Often, spouses whose relationship has deteriorated accumulate a whole list of complaints against each other. But endless complaints will get us nowhere. Before we start making changes, we must thoroughly ponder our priorities, consider the limited mental budget of our partner, select the item that is our highest priority – and change it. We should not complain or give orders. The most we can do is to formulate a request or provide a stimulus by stating a given fact.

"I really want to go to the exhibition at the museum. Would you like to join me?"

He might say yes, and he might say no. If you give up the idea, you will not make any change. Suppose you do not give up. You go to the museum with a male friend who likes art and enjoys your company and you both have a good time there. And you should probably choose a male friend. You need to make your husband realize that he has missed a potentially enjoyable activity with his wife and that another man benefited from it. If you go with a girlfriend or with your sister, he might not have any regrets. Why should he? He is off the hook. Let his wife find something to do with herself. It is as if you went to another room to read a book. But if you go to the museum with a male friend, perhaps after a while your husband will become interested in art exhibitions.

I wish to emphasize again that you should not generalize from the examples I provide. These recommendations are not suitable for everyone. Each case should be examined separately, and only then should you decide how to proceed. If the spouse of the art lover is a fine husband with only one or two limitations, perhaps his wife should not impose a burden on a relationship that is otherwise wonderful, since she has something to lose.

Sometimes one partner takes action to make his or her life easier, but such steps will not improve the relationship. An example of such a change is a case where the woman finds a lover. The implication is that she is investing her efforts elsewhere, instead of enriching her relationship. Her husband, who is forced to deal with the new situation, might relieve his suffering by befriending another woman. Such a friendship might even make the wife stop taking him for granted and reinvest in their marriage so as to save it from total destruction.

Finally, it is important to know that it is always better to start change at home and turn elsewhere only if we are convinced that the situation is hopeless. If you cannot enjoy your own husband, how do you know that you can enjoy someone else? Turning to a man who is not your husband might fail, since you do not have the tools to enjoy him. At the same time, it might ruin your marriage. On the other hand, learning to enjoy your husband might save your marriage, but even if it does not, it will equip you with a new tool that will assist you in building a new relationship in the future. That's why it is always recommended to make the most of an existing relationship, and only if this cannot be done, to seek solutions elsewhere.

Rachel – A case study

Rachel's story, similar to the others described in this book, does not present a solution for all women whose husbands cheat. Each case must be examined separately; nevertheless, it is an interesting and inspiring tale.

Rachel, a married woman and the mother of two, found out recently that her husband, a businessman, had a lover. Rachel came to see me after she realized her husband knew that she knows and was about to move out. A brief interview made me realize that Rachel was a wonderful woman. She had a full-time job and functioned well as a homemaker and mother. Her husband used to go on business trips, and she believed that had he spent more time at home, he would have invested more in his wife and children.

I refused to put all the blame on him. In my opinion, Rachel, by letting herself be taken for granted and allowing him to be away from home frequently, had contributed to a situation in which her husband had capabilities in areas in which she was limited. I asked her how many men she had been with besides her husband. As you might guess, he was the first and only man in her life, which means he had abilities she had not developed yet. Another woman, with a different cocktail of abilities, might have taken advantage of the fact that she had such a "convenient" husband who was often away and had love affairs in ideal conditions. Her husband might then have realized that he must devote more time and energy to her in order to save his marriage. It is as if Rachel had told him: "I am yours no matter what, waiting for you like a piece of furniture." She simply let her husband off the hook. Other than that, the only way she expressed her dissatisfaction was through various complaints, which are naturally the best way to alienate a spouse.

Rachel could seize the opportunity and divorce her husband, keep some of the assets, get her alimony and move on without him, or she could try to save the marriage. In any case, she had to make a drastic change in herself, especially if she wanted to try to salvage the relationship. She had to change drastically so that her husband would not recognize the new Rachel.

During the first meeting I learned two more things about her: She said she was allergic to dust and, although she had a driver's license, she was driven to my office by a friend since she did not drive out of town. When I asked her why she limited herself this way, she said she was afraid of the wheel. I told her I would not let her limit her mobility any more, especially since her husband was so mobile, and that she must drive herself to our next meeting.

"But, I can't!"

"You can. You just don't feel like it."

I asked her what would have happened if her children were injured and needed to be driven to the hospital urgently. Would she wait for someone else to come and drive them?

"I would drive them myself, but I would be very frightened."

"You can drive really slowly and take a break every kilometer or two. If you can't do a minor task like driving a car, how can you possibly handle a much more sophisticated task such as the marital crisis you are going through?"

As for her sensitivity to dust – I suggested a change here too. I asked her to try cautiously to ignore this sensitivity and stay in dusty places. When a person defines himself as allergic, he is usually told to avoid the source of allergy. Avoiding a common element such as dust weakens the person, since it forces him to live in a sort of sterile bubble. When adopting friendly thinking, it is recommended to check whether it is a real allergy or just an oversensitivity which was nurtured with time and was finally classified as a medical problem. If dust does not constitute real mortal danger, but rather an inconvenience which can be dealt with easily, perhaps it is better for us to expose ourselves to it.

In addition to these tasks, I asked Rachel to meet a friend of mine, a lawyer, in order to get some legal guidance, just for the sake of learning. She was not supposed to make a decision regarding any legal steps, but rather to learn about the status of the children and the property.

The next time we met, Rachel arrived much earlier and seemed very happy. It turned out she decided to drive, left the house early, and realized after driving for a few minutes on the highway that the fear had gone and she could enjoy herself.

Rachel told me that during the meeting with the lawyer she learned that she could easily divorce her husband and keep some of the property and money. At this stage she said she was interested in saving her marriage. However, it was good for her to know that she had other options. At the end of the meeting I gave her some even more difficult homework: I told her to initiate relationships with other men.

During the next few weeks Rachel started managing her life in a way that made her days more fulfilling and her time with her children more enjoyable. She went off on weekends with her children to the south and to the north, and for the first time she invited men to her bed. Some of them were even more handsome than her husband.

Rachel's husband did not know about the other men, but he witnessed the evolution of a different woman and started courting her passionately. He moved back in and ended his affair. But Rachel was not in a hurry to go back to the old relationship. She went out with him occasionally, but went out without him as well. She went on trips and even flew abroad without him. By the way, even her sensitivity to dust vanished as if it had never existed.

Six months later her relationship with her husband resembled an ongoing honeymoon. I believe that even today, years after our sessions together, her husband is still waiting for her to come back from her numerous activities, and she even keeps in touch with one or two of her male pals.

Change for couples – When they are not best buddies

Relationships are not a humdrum, routine journey free of crises and shifts. Quarrels, ennui, affairs, rifts between spouses when only one of the partners continues to develop, children leaving home, and many other factors produce a need to make changes in a relationship. An example of such a shift, which is actually a joyful event, is the birth of a first child. Often, after giving birth for the first time, the mother devotes all her mental budget to the new baby and to adjusting to a new, expanded identity. Such a situation changes the relationship since the mother invests part of the mental budget, which was previously invested in her partner, in the demanding infant.

When the mother and her partner are good friends, the shift is not made at the expense of the relationship. On the contrary, it is as if both partners move on to the next grade as they become parents. The spouse stands by her at all times, supports her, helps her, substitutes for her when she is tired, and is just as excited and enthusiastic with the new addition to the family. He does not feel that the baby interferes, but that the baby adds a new layer to his identity. Usually the father is busy with his work during the day, while the mother takes care of the baby in the very first months of life, and a certain shift in the relationship does take place. However, within a few weeks, the identity of both partners already includes parenthood, and they start spending time together again as a couple. Thus, they are on their way to becoming a friendly family.

Such a friendly scenario is not common to all couples following the birth of the first child, but it is definitely possible. In our learning culture it could be achieved rather pleasantly and easily. After a short period of adjustment, the mental abilities of both spouses recover. Their world expands and enables them to include both the new baby and each other.

The example I chose to give – the birth of the first child – is a rather easy shift. Most times it occurs in a period when the spouses are not jaded and are still willing to invest in each other. In addition it is an external event, obvious and definite, unlike other changes that take place slowly and which are often difficult to notice. For these reasons, it is easy enough to make the necessary changes after the birth of the first child.

However, in most other situations, it is not easy to make changes in a relationship. The sense of belonging, which is an important component of a relationship, ties both partners to their old habits. If there are rifts between the spouses, the person who continues to develop has the opportunity of making change, but will succeed only by managing to let go of the aspect of belonging. In fact, the developing partner must upset the balance of the relationship and even be willing to be the "bad guy."

Maria, whose husband got depressed after being fired from his workplace, did exactly that. At first, all the members of the family were affected by his moods and walked on eggshells in order not to hurt his feelings. Maria, who understood the need for change, tried to convince her husband to go out with her from time to time. She suggested many options and tried to initiate change that included him. However, Maria's suggestions were invariably rejected. Eventually, she decided not to give up on her own life. She found various pleasurable activities and enjoyed herself without her husband. Soon she started to live again. She worked, went out to have fun, took care of the children and behaved as if she were a single parent.

Maria's story is an extreme example. Before reaching such a conclusion, one should consider the expected implications, especially if the husband is in the midst of a crisis. In this particular case, it is unclear how Maria's behavior will affect her husband. If he pulls himself together and make changes, they will move on to the next grade together. If he remains behind, he might lose his wife.

When change is made by couples who have been together for many years, it can follow two opposite courses. We have discussed the friendly course in which both spouses make a decision together and act upon it quite easily. For instance, they decide to learn dancing and overnight become the main attraction of every party. They look like professional dancers, and it does not even matter who initiated the change. After a while one of them suggests trying a new position in bed, and the other spouse welcomes the suggestion. Mutual decisions are powerful and can lead to amazing success.

Even when the reason for change is some kind of problem, if both spouses decide to act to improve their relationship, making change is easy. They both take measures to enhance the quality of pleasurable time they spend together, using techniques of cultural management and sexual innovation. The problem they once shared seems smaller or even disappears altogether.

However, a number of relationships are change-resistant. Often, even when both partners agree they must solve a certain problem, they still present a solid united front in totally resisting change. I, the person whose job it is to promote change and advance their relationship, sometimes experience immense frustration, tear my hair out and give up.

In other cases, one partner attempts to make a change, while the other partner blocks the way. The one who wants to make the change must be extremely determined to pursue change when the other spouse is always interfering. The other spouse is not always aware of the interference. Sometime they claim they are ready for the change and even believe it, but in practice, they act against it. If I believe the change is indeed a friendly one, I try to support the activist partner as much as I can. Like an acrobat in the circus, I find myself siding with the husband who wants to leave the small-city apartment and move to the country, and do whatever I can to assist him, while, at other times, I may side with the wife who wishes to complete her academic studies.

I allot two or three meetings to couples who do not change. Sometimes I manage to make them cooperate. One method is to scare them by indicating something that might happen to them if they do not change. An example might be that one of their adolescent children will want to cut all ties with them. When they hear such predictions, they sometimes wake up and cooperate. When there is cooperation, the process of making change is amazing. It is also true in the case of spouses who are at odds with each other and who hate and attack each other. Success in such cases can be achieved by performing the bypass drill: the two of them need, at this stage, to bypass the essence of their conflict and act together creatively.

During the first stages of the change process, the couple is asked to prepare lists giving information about themselves, each describing him or herself. They write about activities they currently share and activities they used to share. In the next stage, they are asked to submit proposals for a future agenda and to think about leisure-time interests they might enjoy together as a couple.

We prepare a schedule for the next couple of days. First, we deal with activities that can be done even when the spouses do not like each other, such as going to the theater. An intimate evening at home by candlelight is not a good idea at this stage. Engaging in sex is a possible activity. I do not mean affectionate loving sex, since the two do not even like each other, but rather quick, purposeful sexual release.

Conversations are not recommended at this stage, because they could rapidly turn into quarrels and hostility. Often I tell such couples that their chances would be better if I could just tape up their mouths like kidnapping victims in the movies. The proverb that says the tongue has the power of life and death is indeed true. It is better for such couples to talk less and do more.

During the next stage, both partners are asked to review their relationship and indicate which points they think the partner has missed out on. According to my view or outlook, I add some items which are not mentioned by either. Now the couples choose a few points from the list to include in their schedule. Some objectives which were previously omitted are now included. Soon they expand their infrastructure of entertainment and enjoyment, and the relationship becomes much more interesting. We can only regret the things they have missed so far, but from now on, they can feel much better than before.

It is important to note that, as always, the content of the homework I give the couple is entirely personal. Each couple should consider the things that are relevant to it. It is important that each partner shows interest in the things the other is interested and those the first partner is unfamiliar with. If, for instance, the husband likes history, and the wife is not drawn to the subject at all, she is ignoring an area which is very significant to him, and that leaves them a very narrow area of common ground. The husband, for his part, may feel justified not to invest in subjects that interest his wife. Just as the abilities of one side trigger the other to learn, so those who decline to learn trigger the other side not to learn. In such a case, the wife's homework would include reading at least five history books. When she gains familiarity with the subject, a new channel will open for the two of them.

Sometimes this is the stage at which the partners finally confront the main controversial issue, the one that bothers them the most. At this stage, when they are less sensitive and upset, there is a chance they will negotiate in a friendly manner even in relation to this controversial issue. In fact, if it is not entirely necessary, I recommend avoiding the crucial subject altogether. It is better for them to devote their efforts to expanding their abilities. They should choose a suitable area in which to gain a new common channel of expression. Such an area could be bridge, played against another couple. Or they could take up computers, dancing or a foreign language. Soon, they may feel that they are on a honeymoon and find it hard to believe that just two months earlier their quarrels were enriching two separate law firms.

Relationships outside marriage – A fling or a love story?

I agree with those who say that a truly great love is worth any price one has to pay. But what is "truly great"?

When it comes to relationships outside marriage, I usually think of them as nothing more than "relationship accidents." I see the widespread cause of road accidents: a slight distraction from the road, and suddenly – a crash. Relations of men and women outside of marriage happen in most cases as a result of neglect, as a minor distraction in the couple's routine. All of a sudden, a chance encounter turns into an affair which morphs into a big messy situation.

I am not claiming that any fling between a man and a woman who are not married to each other is a mess. Millions of people all over the world have friendships outside of marriage. A married woman meets a married man from time to time for short periods. They enjoy each other's company and then return to their own homes, their own worlds and identities. From a certain perspective, it is not that different from playing tennis with a friend without one's partner. But society refers to it differently. And the bombastic term that is used for such encounters is "cheating."

It gets messy when two people who are not single fall in love with each other and decide to leave everything behind and be together. Here, sometimes, we can find one of the most dangerous and sophisticated means of rejection disguised as falling in love. It is not a friendly act but a destruction of everything that was previously built. It is difficult to present it as such to the new couple. They are captivated by their emotions and unable to see the big picture. So when they finally sober up, everything around them is already ruined and destroyed.

Zachary, a rich contractor, fell in love with a young woman who worked at his office. They had an exciting but incomplete relationship. They started to feel they wanted to become more serious. He bought an apartment in the woman's name, got divorced and was about to move in with his lover. However, on the very day he moved in with her, she became emotionally paralyzed, lost all interest in him and could not stand his touch. She wanted him to leave at once. So, after burning all bridges, Zachary found himself alone. He had lost both his lover and his wife.

On the other hand, Sami, a mother of three, reached a stage of total depression with regard to her marriage of 18 years, which had been unbalanced for a long time. Her husband, "a good guy" in the negative sense of the words, was a classic example of one who declines to learn and remains with his limited abilities. She, on the other hand, became independent and full of life and desired to move forward. At a certain point she got in touch with a divorced man and after a few months of an incomplete but enjoyable relationship, she decided not to make do with the occasional meetings but to exchange her husband for the new man. The transformation involved great distress. Some of the children did not accept the drastic move, and it took two years until a friendly relationship was formed between them and the new partner. Today, ten years later, it seems that Sami has made a friendly change. Her former husband also moved on. He became friends with another woman and enjoys his relationship with her much more than the one he had with his ex-wife.

How can one know if ending the old relationship and building a new one is a wise move? People who are part of the relationship cannot answer this question. In such a case, each one has to ask and sincerely answer a few blunt questions. Often I find myself introducing these questions. It is not easy to talk to a person in love who is carried away by emotions. Such people find it difficult to see the scenery and are aware only of their passions. Facts cannot distract them from their emotions.

Sam had an affair with Michelle. Michelle was married to his business partner, and both Michelle and Sam had young children. The love between them flourished. However, from my perspective, I saw only destruction. Sam was on the verge of making a major deal, a once-in-a-lifetime opportunity which would be canceled if the affair was exposed. I saw the affair as a crude rejection of the business opportunity. Eventually Sam decided the affair was like gunpowder that might blow up everything he had built. He promised not to meet his lover again. I warned him that it might be extremely difficult and that he might fail since forced restraint could lead to an explosion. I suggested that instead of investing all his energies on avoiding her, he should fill up his days with activities that were new, enriching and entertaining. He chose to invest in his wife, his children and sports. It was a worthy investment, and the relationship with Michelle faded away.

A compound family

People who are married for the second or third time have special problems. When the woman is divorced with two children, the man is divorced with one child, and they have a baby together, the relationship is bound to be affected by the relationship of the man with the woman's children, the relationship of the woman with the man's child, and sometimes even by the relationship with the ex-husband or ex-wife. There are many other similar scenarios.

In such a case, the children represent popular opinion. Too many people are oppressed by their children and allow them to decide whether to accept or reject a particular companion. Friendships that depend entirely on the children's whims are doomed to fail. Many such friendships explode unpleasantly. In other such friendships, the couple does not make the most of the relationship. They live separately, focus on their own children and meet each other from time to time. Their relationship only stands a chance if the couple puts it in the center and takes the children along, at first one-by-one, and gradually all of them. The children who are called to join in are the children who accept the new partner and do not pose a threat to the relationship. If one particular child is hostile towards the new partner and rejects him or her, it is better to relegate this child to the perimeter and invest in the other children. Such an investment might, with time, encourage this child to join the others.

Staying together at any price?

I am not the guru of family relationships, and I do not believe family always comes first. Sometimes, such an attachment is, in fact, a restriction – those involved might feel as if they are suffocating in a dungeon. If such is the case, we need to set them free. Nevertheless, I am not hasty when it comes to divorce. The following sentence contradicts what many people feel and believe: normally, **it is better not to start a new relationship before checking out whether we have overlooked or missed out on something in a former relationship.** Usually, it is much more economical to freshen up an old relationship with a friendly foundation than to go back to square one in order to build something new. Such a beginning means moving sideways instead of forwards. The energy devoted to the new relationship will take us to a point we have already been at. This axiom is not always true, but before people decide to get a divorce, it is better for them to think carefully whether they have taken advantage of everything the former relationship offered, and whether they are moving forward to a better place. Perhaps these people are just stuck, and ending the relationship would cause them to miss some things they did not sufficiently appreciate in the previous relationship.

Occasionally, when I ask partners to prepare a list of personal abilities together with a list that includes their abilities as a couple, the different lists show a huge gap between the impressive abilities of each partner and those abilities they share as a couple. The man's list includes various interesting occupations, and the woman's list includes many hobbies, but the lists are separate and entirely different. One can see that they live side-by-side, each of them leading an interesting life, but their shared sphere is narrow and neglected. They make do with their framework as a couple without considering or investing in the qualitative quotient of their joint time. Such a relationship is extremely shaky, as it is very easy to demolish it. Both partners might find themselves enjoying somebody else's company – somebody with shared abilities.

Such missed opportunities are very common. When I ask the man why he did not accompany his wife to the dance class one evening, he says bluntly: "I don't like to dance." This means he does not know how to dance, because a person who knows how to dance always enjoys it, and it also means he has never bothered to learn. Conversely, when I ask the woman why she wasn't curious about her husband's business, she says: "I am not interested in that."

Examining the situation with a friendly view or outlook reveals that she is paying a high price for her lack of interest – her husband prefers to share this central part of his identity with other people.

On the other hand, if she does not bother to become interested in 12th-century music which he listens to once or twice a year – it is not that bad. It would not hurt her to expand her knowledge of medieval music, but even if she doesn't, her family will not collapse.

I definitely do not believe that partners are supposed to do everything together. Even if they know how to make the most of themselves as a couple and produce the things they are able to produce together, each of them still has unique capabilities. The husband would express them without the wife and vice versa. However, when too many things are done separately, the relationship is neglected. Sometimes the couple had interesting and exciting time together in the past but then starts to neglect their relationship, usually because of other intensive pressures.

In light of all this, when partners announce their intention to divorce, I try first to promote mutual productive activities. Usually, the spouses cooperate, succeed and decide to stay together. But even if they decide to go their own separate ways, a friendly mutual production increases chances of reaching a friendly separation agreement based on cooperation.

We all change throughout our lives, and sometimes a man and a woman who once fit together do not suit one another anymore. It might be because one of them changed, while the other remained the same, or because each of them has moved in a different direction. Sometimes the gaps are so huge that a separation seems friendlier than a reunion.

An example of such a case is a couple which starts out religious, but a few years later, one of them becomes less observant. Normally, the one who is more limited, anf finds the rules of religion too restrictive, imposes curbs on the other's behavior. If, for instance, the man is the one who becomes less religious, he will try not to eat ham or violate the Sabbath when his wife is around. But the wife might be extremely concerned about the possibility that he might eat ham elsewhere or break the Sabbath when he is not with her. In such a case, perhaps there is no other option but to separate, because the price that each is required to pay to be considerate towards the other is much too high.

Another example of a change that in most cases will lead to the end of the relationship is a woman telling her husband: "I do not want us to separate, but I also love Alex and want to be with him from time to time."
I would inform this woman that there are many types of relationships: exclusive relationships, exclusive relationships with hidden "extras"' love triangles, partner-swapping for fun and so on. But if there is no symmetry, and one is enjoying life while the other one is suffering- there are only two options: to give up the affair or to split up the couple. Some women might conceal their affairs, and some husbands might even accept the condition, but usually the husband feels he cannot continue in such a relationship and prefers to end it.

These are only two examples of unsymmetrical changes. Usually the one that has the ability leads the way, and if the spouse is unable to change, the rift between the two widens. Eventually the one who is able and capable moves on with life, leaving behind the more limited partner.

***

The husband-wife unit and the basic family unit are undergoing great changes these days, after being stable for centuries. Nowadays, more people have the ability to end the relationship. I will dare to ask a question that nobody likes to hear: isn't it true that a long-lasting relationship may reflect the limitations of partners who remain on the same level, do not make any changes, and are unable to leave each other even if they do not enjoy each other anymore? Sometimes, it is indeed true.

To sum up this chapter, let us go back to the couples with the wonderful capabilities discussed in the beginning of the chapter, the ones who have long-lasting friendships and love each other, and whose mutual enjoyment improves with time. If we listen to these capable people, we will find out that they keep enjoying each other because they constantly renew their relationships. They go on "honeymoons" and keep their close connection alive. Maintaining consistency is highly important, since in light of the numerous stimuli out there, neglect is our worst enemy and can destroy a relationship in no time.

Chapter 10

Change in Sex Life – From a Kitten to a Tiger

Sex – Do not settle for a little

Even though sex is one of the most discussed topics in Western culture, its importance in relationships does not always get the attention it deserves.

Partners respond to each other. Sometimes they are both turned on at the same moment, but usually it does not happen this way. One of them desires the other, expresses desire, sometimes implicitly; the other is turned on a few seconds later, and they both enjoy each other. It is not important who initiates the act. A single initiator is enough.

Sex and physical contact in general are very important parts of friendship. In addition, since sex is a sensitive topic in our society, it sometimes serves as part of the change process even when the change required is in a completely different area. For instance, when a husband who was once a salaried employee becomes self-employed and his wife starts working with him, they have to make a lot of changes together and separately. But soon they realize that in order to work well as a team, they must also consider their sexual relationship. The existing pattern is somewhat burdensome and involves anger and bad moods. It is clear that they have to change this pattern so it will not stand in the way of other changes.

There are ways to help us make changes in this area: various positions, new locations besides the bed, music, different lighting – such as candlelight – as well as a vibrator, Viagra or group sex. Other than that, it is important to get to know one's body and its abilities and to focus on one's partner through the senses. All of these can magically improve our sex lives.

Task: Senses and sensuality

When we are in bed with a partner, even when it is a one-time fling, we should focus on our partner exclusively. By doing that we will increase our own enjoyment. To distinguish between what is important and what is less important, we must learn how to focus our senses on a person or an object we are interested in and not let others distract us. Let us practice using our senses in our daily lives:

Sense of sight: Look at something like a tree branch, a bird, a plate of food, the woman by our side. The aim is to train the brain to focus on a certain object chosen by the sense of sight. In other words, looking at the plate, the branch, or the partner, without thinking about something else at the same time. Our thoughts wander? Focus again on the object. We cannot go on? Leave it and try again later.

Sense of hearing: Close your eyes to avoid other stimuli and concentrate primarily on noises around you: music, sounds from the street, birds chirping, the sound of wind, a woman's breathing. And again, focus on the sounds around.

Practice with the other senses as well. When in bed with a partner – we should feel her body and concentrate on her skin, the softness of her hair, her stomach, the smell of her body. Close your eyes and focus on her taste.

Just as when learning to play the piano we practice with our right hand at first, and then with our left hand, and only then play with both hands, this should be the pattern here. We should invest time and practice until our brain is able to focus on the input of several senses at the same time. After practicing with the senses, one will be able to smell a lover's hair, feel the touch of her hands on his skin, and listen to the sounds she makes all at the same time. Concentrating on the senses blocks all interference and increases the ability to enjoy the act of love.

The twelfth night – from platonic friendship to sexual endeavor

When we wish to check whether we can become a couple, we can start from a cultural, intellectual and social production and finally add friendship in bed. On our way, we might face difficulties since it is not easy to move from platonic friendship to sexual endeavor.

Many of us believe that we can't go to bed with a person that we don't have a crush on, and even if we are willing to try, the trial usually reinforces the impression we had beforehand. This means that most of us are victims of our own prejudices. We should do ourselves a favor and make a sensual, friendly change in this area as well. Though at first it is not easy, we should make an effort. We should not wait until we feel a burning desire before we act. If we add sexual enjoyment to the equation, we will benefit from it. Perhaps we will start enjoying ourselves only on the twelfth night? So what – it is worth it!

Why should we relate sexually to people who do not arouse us at first? Because people who are able to go to bed only with people whom they find extremely attractive limit themselves. Many people become "enslaved" to the people they got used to, and do not try to do it with others, who could turn out to be good friends. They are stuck and make do with almost nothing. In practice, they do not have any freedom of choice. If one can manage to enjoy sex even without that initial attraction, one is empowered to choose the best partner.

Another important argument is that even people who have regular partners find it difficult to sustain intense sexual enjoyment throughout the years. Many of them experience a dry spell in bed. The learners overcome the problem easily, and the ones whose learning tools are less developed feel bad since their level of desire has changed. They might settle for very little and lose some of their joy of life or experience stormy periods in their lives – for instance, become involved in destructive affairs. For this reason, we should deal with erotic fluctuations and not let them dictate our agenda exclusively.

Male–Female – Find the differences

When a man and a woman are about to start a course of sexual renewal, which they can manage by themselves or with a little external help, it is important for them to be aware of each other.

The man should identify his partner's ability, know how to please her and understand her reactions. The woman should do the same for the man.

When such people come to see me, I hold separate sessions with each of them. People tend not to speak openly about such subjects when their partners are in the room. In this session I ask what they have produced together, identify the things they have missed and review the gap between their personal ability and their mutual productivity. In many such sessions, the gaps between women and men with regard to the way they perceive sex are shown. Their expectations from their partners in bed are different, their perceptions about what is allowed and what is forbidden are different. The importance they attach to sex is different. In addition, we must consider the obvious physical differences which are responsible for the fact that the pace of their arousal is different and their manner of reaching satisfaction is different.

Sandra and Jacob, who were in their thirties and had two young children, led an unsatisfactory sex life. Throughout the years Jacob has felt humiliated and sexually frustrated. He wanted sex frequently, while Sandra felt she did not like sex. Occasionally, after Jacob nagged time and time again, Sandra "did him a favor." I did not accept the argument that he was very eager and she was frigid. I believed they had created a situation which enabled Jacob to be, in his own eyes, a man with "healthy male urges" and Sandra to perceive herself as a desirable woman. In fact she served him by refusing him, by letting him be sexually aroused for a long period of time.

When I met Jacob alone, I told him he was not allowing his wife to desire him since he expressed his lust non-stop. I suggested that he reach sexual satisfaction in different ways. It would enable him to be less sexually interested in Sandra, and it might make her more interested in him.

In meetings at which both spouses are present, I sometimes tell the woman something I want the man to hear, and I make her say something I actually want the man to listen to. So at our next meeting, when Sandra was also present, I said out loud that Jacob could always be with another woman. I noticed how Sandra became alert when she heard this.

When I met Sandra in private, I suggested that she not wait until she felt a burning desire, but make a decision to become eager and act upon it, otherwise she might lose her husband. I mentioned that the option I presented to her husband might actually be utilized. If he truly believed his wife did not want him, he might someday meet someone who desired him, and one thing would lead to another. I added that, contrary to what she believed, she was able to have more sex than any man in the world. Finally, I emphasized that she could easily change the pattern – all she had to do was to initiate sex, day after day.

"That's what he wants. It won't change a thing. He will be pleased and ask for more."

I suggested that after she initiated sex, when he wanted to get some sleep, she should initiate another round, and another – until he rejects her because he is not able to proceed. The thought that he is not able to respond to his wife's proposal would be very unpleasant. In addition, I asked her to think seriously about the topic of abilities. I told her that there is no doubt men are more sexually limited than women. A professional prostitute can even serve a few dozen men a night. No man is capable of that. In her mind's eye, Sandra attached such an ability to Jacob, whereas, in fact, she was the one with the ability.

Sandra did as I said and discovered that she could initiate sex. She enjoyed her new ability and probably would never agree to go back to the previous pattern that limited her so much.

Tit and tallit – A case study

Mike and Shelly were two Americans who immigrated to Israel as young adults. They had a religious education, were considered "good children" and got married at a young age. They were both scientists and very busy with their work. They did not have many friends and, most importantly, they did not have a sex life. They claimed not to be bothered by the situation, but the fact that after five years of marriage they were still childless bothered them.

When they came to see me it turned out that they had tried in vain to have sexual intercourse several times. Erectile problems may be caused by repressed homosexual tendencies or other reasons. Shelly, who expected her husband to function as a man, was hurt, thinking he was not attracted to her. At other times he was ready to do it, but she was too dry. Without talking much about it, they had a silent agreement to avoid the whole ordeal of sexual relations. If it wasn't for the pressure put on them by religious society to have children, they might have continued to live like that forever.

First, I advised them to avoid one-time encounters that make them feel like failures. At this stage, they could not possibly manage a spectacular experience of having sexual intercourse and getting pregnant. They still had not developed the necessary ability, and they lacked the tools to reach their goal. First they must learn how to perform and create a certain infrastructure that would enable them at a later stage to break through the barrier of shame which had forced them to be stuck at the same point for such a long time.

Obviously, the fact that they were both religious limited their ability to make cultural changes. For that reason, each was asked to prepare a personal list of shame barriers in other domains of life, not necessarily in sex, and a list of suggestions of "bold" changes in various domains.

Shelly's lists included suggestions such as singing out loud in front of an open window so that the neighbors could hear (strict Jewish tradition views a woman's solo singing as seductive); wearing colorful clothes; going out without her wig; being late to work. Mike also wrote about wearing colorful clothes as well as other acts: leaving work in the middle of the day; praying at home on Sabbath instead of praying at the synagogue and sometimes not praying at all; enjoying sports, including bungee-jumping. We prepared a common list to which I added an item – watching pornographic movies together and separately. Then I asked Mike if he was willing to take off his yarmulke just to go into a sex shop to buy a vibrator, or whether he would like me to buy it for him. He preferred to do it himself. I asked Shelly whether she would prefer to talk to a woman about intimate issues rather than to talk to me. She blushed and said she preferred to face this difficulty with me. Later I asked her if she would agree not to wear her bra occasionally, and I asked them to start doing some physical exercises such as walking or dancing, which were not customary in their community.

Within days they were both euphoric. They had a secret which was theirs alone and perceived themselves as partners in crime. They started having fun and laughing a lot. Every day brought something new that freshened up their lives. She started singing out loud in front of open windows, and he sometimes joined her with his slightly rusty voice. They started jogging at night, took up dancing, bought colorful clothes for Mike and sexy underwear for Shelly – and when they bought them, Mike actually went into the shop with the skullcap on his head. In addition they chose a few pornographic movies and watched them together. In short, they started stimulating themselves and their dormant relationship.

I have no idea which of the above was the most beneficial, but after a while they came to see me with shining eyes and told me they now had a regular sex life. A few months later I heard Shelly was pregnant.

***

Usually I do not easily dismiss making changes related to a couple's sex life. Refusal to learn is the only reason to interrupt this process. Nevertheless, there were also cases of couples who convinced me they were rarely interested in sex. Since both spouses wanted only infrequent sex, they were still friends in bed. I suggested they did not change this arrangement but perceive it as a position they both felt comfortable with. It was important, though, to free themselves from the negative feelings attached to it. Spouses need to find a suitable formula that works for them and makes their sex life enjoyable and fulfilling.

Chapter 11

Change with Children – Growing with the Child

Children as friends

Many parents pass on to their children not only the wisdom and experience they have gained over the years, but also an assortment of nonsense inherited from previous generations. In fact, many children fail to develop fully their abilities, identities, and especially their freedom of thought partly because of their mom and dad. Most of them get into traditional, unfriendly grooves that are shaped by their parents and teachers. At a certain point their brains become blocked, and from then on the children only repeat themselves in the most predictable way. Children have a miraculous learning ability until we grownups interfere and suppress it.

The diagnostic culture, which is very harmful to grownups, is even more devastating where young children are concerned. Most people believe that the sooner they detect problematic symptoms, the better. But if, instead of keeping their eyes on their children's developing abilities, parents constantly lie in wait for their failures, they risk shaping the child's identity as problematic. Young children form their identity almost entirely through the way in which adults see them. For this reason, relating to children only by way of their problems is, in my opinion, a serious fault.

Friendly parents acknowledge their own abilities and limitations and do not present themselves as omnipotent. In addition, they will notice the growing abilities of their children, which the latter should enjoy and add to their expertise. Instead of serving the children's **needs**, which only encourages limitations and unnecessary dependence, they will serve their **growth** and nurture their talents. This way they will avoid the crude, fixed pattern so many parents develop. They will be glad to see that their 10-year-old son swims better than his mom and dad or is more computer literate than them, and be happy that he still enjoys his parents' company. The parents in turn will teach him how to include them and his siblings in his life and how to maintain normative relations with them. The child will learn various social combinations which will broaden his horizons and expand his emotional experiences. He will know the difference between being independent and on his own and being around other human beings who deserve consideration.

Many times it is not necessary to drag children to therapy. Parents can easily produce change in their children if it is required. This way, the main part of raising children will be enjoying family life and not a heavy load of responsibilities and exhausting services. Many parents miss out on enjoyment and believe that a necessary part of raising children is bearing a heavy burden on their shoulders.

Moreover, we will soon clarify how children can do an excellent job of teaching their parents how to change. With their help, the parents too will be able to develop and move ahead.

Task: Changing the routine

Normally it is recommended that children have a fixed schedule, since it provides security and stability. However, although routine has its merits, if we want a child who is not just a follower and conformist, we can change a routine from time to time. Children who are only used to fixed patterns will acquire an unwanted, unfriendly mental limitation which will make it hard for them to fulfill their potentials. For this reason, it is a positive move to take children on an outing or to the bowling alley in the middle of the school week.

In fact, the ability to change a routine is important at any age. In order to become open to change, we should know how to disrupt arbitrarily the most inflexible habits. If our weekends follow a fixed pattern, and they probably do, we should introduce a deliberate change: one weekend we may go to the beach, and the next weekend we may watch TV most of the time. On the third weekend we might decide to stay in a hotel. Similarly, from time to time, we should include foods which we are not used to in our dinner menus, visit new places, and generally spice up our daily routine.

We have a baby

The birth of the first child starts a couple on a completely new track. The baby has immediate needs which cannot be postponed. It must be fed and soothed 24/7. When the baby is sick or in pain, the parents stay awake all night, and the question "Whose turn is it to get up now?" is raised repeatedly. Other weighty questions come up as well. Some parents try to avoid tasks, while others carry them out readily. Generally speaking, the arrival of the firstborn with its constant demands challenges the parents' egocentrism. Until now, this couple was focused on themselves and on their relationship. However, a true learner learns quickly. Most adults are equipped to give the baby everything it needs, and the difficulties ease off within a few weeks. The parents' world gradually expands and is now able to include others.

The baby is capable of exerting a certain influence on the parents which cannot be applied by anybody else, and by doing so, it forces them to move on to the next stage. Let us consider a new mother who was not interested in change. If the young father is interested in change, she might break up with him. If her own mother urges her to change, she might minimize contact with her. But the baby can do the impossible and dictate change. From now on she must take care of her child, and the child's appearance on the scene is not a one-time event. The baby is there to stay. Thus, babies are an excellent impetus for change, almost the best there is.

The first nights of new parents are difficult. Later on, even if they experience a difficult night from time to time, they are capable of handling it. They continue to develop on a daily basis, and new components are added to their world. By becoming parents they undergo an unequivocal identity change. They will never be kids again. From now on, there is another human being in the center of their identity. Almost all important steps in their lives will include this small human being.

Almost all of us reach the stage at which we are required to meet our child's needs, but some people become stuck in this phase. If we do not continue to develop, we will miss a great deal. In fact, babies grow up quick as lightning. The phase in which the baby is totally dependent on the parent is very short. An infant's ability develops steadily, and in a short while, they can do many things independently.

The child is growing. How about us?

Babies become toddlers and then preschoolers rather quickly. Are we aware of the changes they go through? Many parents are only equipped with the necessary tools to take care of a baby. When they have an infant, mom and dad know exactly what to do, whether it be carrying the infant or changing diapers. Now, when they have a young child, they continue this familiar pattern. They serve another term dressing the child and doing laundry, and the child adjusts to their limitations.

A good relationship between parents and children does not mean we need to meet the children's needs but to nurture their growth. Being with your child should not be a task, but a pleasant experience. That is why we should include the child in activities that interest us. When children notice we are having fun, they will meet us at our best. Our enjoyment affects the child, and the result is a friendly deal. If, for instance, the mother likes to watch football matches on TV, her children will get excited as well even if they don't understand the essence of the game. We must remember that, at this stage, we are the ones teaching our children about reality.

As parents, we must follow two important rules. First, we must be aware of our abilities and recognize our available mental budget, which means knowing when we are at our best, and when we are not, and making sure we are at our best in the presence of the child. Parents who do that soon find out that they are much more pleased with themselves, and the process which seemed constraining quickly becomes an identity change.

The second important rule is not to misread the ability of the child who is constantly growing and developing. By the time we finally learn what to do with a three-year-old, he is already four years old. We do not always manage to keep track of the rapid pace of development, and sometimes we have an *idée fixe* of our children at a particular age in our minds. We must constantly update our conceptualization and change our repertoire of cultural activities and entertainment accordingly.

Seeing the world through the eyes of a child – The smell of the ground after rain

When we, as parents, need to integrate the child into our world, we should not arrogate to ourselves talents which are not included in our repertoire, but we should, of course, continue to expand our world. We should take advantage of the fact that we have a young child and bond with him or her. We then will be able to experience things we forgot a long time ago. When was the last time we noticed an anthill? We should look at the anthill through the eyes of our child and notice how interesting it is. Growing with our child gives us the opportunity to smell the ground after rain, to hear the whispers of the wind, and to transform what we may consider junk into a magical world. We should take our children along to activities we enjoy and connect them to activities they enjoy the most. Children are able to restore some of our lost curiosity. A young child is an awesome learner, at least until grownups take away the pleasure of learning.

It is important to observe the world from our children's height, to accompany our children and mediate between them and the unfolding world. The child gives us an opportunity to avoid mistakes made when we were children, which affected the way we perceived the world. When I was a little boy, my friends and I thought that applying mud to a wound improved the healing process. When I did that, it caused a severe infection. I have grown up and taught my own children about various medicines and their purpose. Another example: parents who did not obtain enough affection as children tend to hug their children a lot. People who heard their parents insult one another make sure they do not do that in front of their children. They are aware of their audience. As parents we face the world of childhood again, only this time we are equipped with more developed tools than the ones we had as children. We should use these tools.

We should also become familiar with new games which will enable us to have fun with our children. However, when we review a book that includes a selection of games, it is important that we do not choose the games we think our child needs, but games that have some entertainment potential for us too. We must remember that if we spend time with our children wearing a bored expression on our faces, we are missing the whole point. If the child sees us weary, exhausted or even desperate, we are not perceived as friends. We diminish the child's enjoyment, because it is not fun to play with someone who does not enjoy the game. Besides that, we are granting the children too much power and misleading them. They might view themselves as Hercules, or a more modern hero like Spiderman.

Such a perception was developed by Danny, five years old, a firstborn with two younger siblings. The parents complained that their son was not disciplined, hit other children in kindergarten and disturbed his teacher. Both parents were educators and had been exposed to all sorts of golden rules about raising children. According to one of these rules, parents should never expose their child to separation anxiety. The parents acted according to this rule, not daring to leave him at home with a babysitter and go out in the evening. By so doing, they granted the child immense power. Danny knew that even if his parents wanted to punish him and not take him on a trip, it would be difficult for them since they would not want to leave him behind. So why should he make an effort and be considerate? Due to fact that Danny's parents were so reluctant to break the rules, they confused their child and enabled him to perceive himself as omnipotent. His perception was reflected in his behavior in kindergarten. Here he even terrorized the teacher, who felt intimidated when dealing with such educated parents.

If we do not interfere with children's development, they will express themselves in a language that suits their ability. They will enjoy expressing their abilities. A person who prevents them from doing so is not a friend. A person who nurtures their weaknesses by encouraging them to remain small hurts them. Neglecting to teach social skills at the right time might weaken the child who will have to deal with the demands of social structures outside the home, such as kindergarten, school, national service and so on. As long as the child does not realize that the rules have distorted his perception of reality, he is doomed to suffer.

However, overprotection is not the only harmful reaction. We must also beware of endless criticism, reproach and yelling. In such a case the children might think that everything they do is awful. If we constantly yell at our children, we might convey the message that they are intrinsically bad. It's very easy for children to take on this role and not so easy to relinquish it.

I have already stressed that we should be at our best when we spend time with our children, at least during their first years of life. These are the years when we influence them the most. We should remember that during this period, we constitute the most reliable source of information for our children.

Starting change

What should we do when our child seems to be throwing off all restraints? As with any other change, we can achieve effective results quickly and easily if we invest in producing maximal ability from all sides and not concentrate only on "the cause" of the problem. Parents do not react inappropriately because they lack ability, but because they lack the necessary knowledge to use it. That is why, first and foremost, we should not be tempted by cheap psychology: the child envies his little brother and this causes his bedwetting; the child needs attention; the child is afraid of the dark — so he develops further anxiety and fears. Such thinking will take us nowhere. Some psychologists who treat children serve as state-of-the-art babysitters. They offer long-term therapy and achieve only partial results. The child returns from the short session with the therapist to the parents with whom he shares his life and who do not change. In fact he is returning to the same environment that produces the symptoms. What good does this do?

There are many different approaches to treating children, and no one approach is suitable for everybody. I believe it is unhelpful to deal with the advantages and disadvantages of a certain approach and important to focus on effectiveness. If someone achieves change and is certain it is due to hanging grapes on his ears, I would certainly encourage him to continue to use this effective method.

I tend to produce change in children, at least till the age of ten, by instructing the parents. The condition is that mom and dad not only live together but are also friends. I do not like the idea of sending young children to psychologists. The parents are the ones with the most clout. The parents, not the therapist, have an opportunity to produce change in their children on a daily basis rather easily, and their chances are much greater than those of a therapist who meets the child once a week. The psychologist can give us advice but cannot treat the child – that is the parents' job.

In addition, I usually do not recommend explicit prohibitions, since they usually turn parents into police officers. Continuing this pattern of unpleasant skirmishes with the child may severely damage the child's identity. If, for instance, we forbid our child to watch TV, and he watches TV when we are not home, he will discover that he has the ability to circumvent the prohibition. Such a perception might get him into trouble later in life. If he can get around his parents' rules, why can't he break the State's laws?

Let us introduce data instead of prohibitions. We should not say: "If you do not behave yourself, we will not take you on our trip," but "On Saturday we are going on a trip with your sister, and you are staying with grandma." We should add an explanation: "We choose to do this because we want to enjoy nature, and we know that if we take you along, it might be unpleasant. When you are older and able to behave appropriately, we will be glad to take you with us." Introducing data is accurate and real – the parents do not prohibit things they can't control. The introduction of data must be consistent, as only then will it lead to change.

Mom and dad or husband and wife

Usually when problematic signs appear, parents rush into treating their child and look for a wonder medicine that will heal him. Sometimes another adult in the child's environment can produce a change without the parents' involvement. An example of such a case might be kindergarten teachers who succeed in weaning children off pacifiers or stops them wetting their pants, while the parents are not able to do so.

However, the best way to produce change in children is to make a family investment, primarily by freshening up the friendship between the spouses. Contrary to common assumptions, the rule of friendly prioritizing does not mean putting the child at the top of the list. A significant part of the parents' mental budget should be devoted to their professional and personal relationships. The child should indeed be a central part of their lives, but at this point in their children's lives, the amount of time we invest in them should be similar to the amount of time we invest in other domains. When we go shopping and our children come along, we invest in them as well as in shopping. When the whole family goes bike riding, both the parents and the children enjoy themselves. As a rule, the number of hours we invest in our child is not the most important thing. Increasing the **duration** of time devoted to our children will not change the situation. Improving the **quality** of the time invested will do the trick.

When the child acts up and we want to produce change, we must start with ourselves. Many parents function as mom and dad and forget about their friendship. They are not aware of the possibility of enjoying one another after their baby has grown. The problematic child saves them the trouble of reinvesting in their friendship. In many cases, when parents are exhausted from their relationship with the child, the father leaves the scene, dedicates himself to his work and lets the mother deal with the children. Obviously, with time, the couple's relationship becomes less solid and they are surrounded by problems which take up most of their time. Mom and dad attack each other and complain about each other at the children's expense. And what happens to the children? The child's symptoms develop. Children are learners. They learn the language of the surroundings created by their parents and react accordingly. Only if the parents are friends will they be a powerful force capable of dealing with most of the children's problems and resolving them.

If the child has become the center of attention at home and we wish to change it, at first we should spend an excessive amount of time outside. If we stay home, it will enable the child to go back to the familiar pattern in which he is the center of the universe, and we will not be strong enough to resist it. Only after we have gathered some strength will we take the child along on some of our outings. But if the child becomes aggressive again, we should reserve the option of leaving him with a babysitter and going out by ourselves again. We should also have a good time with the child one-on-one. After we notice a significant change in our child's behavior, we can start doing pleasurable activities at home. The first layer has been built and stability achieved. The next phase will be easier to implement.

Common language

As a couple who has regained its friendly relationship, we are now ready to form a united strategic front with regard to the child. However, if the child gets mixed signals at home, numerous difficulties will arise. The mother tells the child he is not allowed to play ball in the morning but lets him do so in the evening. The father tells the child he must be a good student, but then allows him to miss a few days of school for a family vacation. Moreover, there are many cases where mom says one thing, while dad says exactly the opposite. Dad tries to set a limit, and mom undermines him. Because the parents are not coordinated, the child gets confused. We must remember: **when it comes to producing change in children, failure is not an option.** Failure might hurt the child throughout life. Success is a must, and building a common strategy is an essential condition.

This strategy includes spending time together. If the father is not around, he does not exist in the child's mind. The child constantly negotiates with the mother, and the father is not perceived as a factor. Consequently the father must show the child that he is part of his world. Once the fatherly presence is established, it will be easier for the father to intervene, while helping the mother and invigorating the system.

Furthermore, you, as the father, are supposed to dedicate some time to your child, to create a meeting point for just the two of you and do something together. In the course of such pastimes, you will be able to create sustainable components of friendship. For instance, if in the future, you ask your child to help his mother and not to burden her, or to behave himself in class, you might produce a certain behavioral change.

I implore mothers to find a more appropriate pastime than talking on and on about bedwetting. How about singing with your children? It is important to know that sometimes, when a woman suppresses her identity to dedicate herself to motherhood and serving her children endlessly, she might find out after her children have grown that they treat her as a servant and do not respect her. Dealing with problems is not the most important thing. If we do not feel that raising our children is fun, it is time to change our perception and enjoy the years when our children are growing. Instead of dwelling on their faults, we should nurture their abilities, develop them and make them our first priority. Obviously, we can make dinner without help, and when our child helps us he makes a mess. So what? At this point we should give priority to the child's ability. In a short while, this ability will improve and the child will be able to make dinner without making a mess – and then it will be time to nurture a new ability.

In addition, it is important for us to be aware of our limitations and not to present ourselves as the sole solution for the child's needs. If we mention that in certain areas the neighbor or an acquaintance is more qualified than us, our child will learn that even if someone else is better than him in certain things, it does not affect his worth. He has already absorbed the fact that there are people who are even more talented than his mom and dad.

For the same reason, we should not claim expertise in everything. We can say: "I do not know the answer to this question. Why don't we look for it together?" Then we should try to find the answer in books, search the Web or ask someone else, and by doing so we will enrich our child's world and our world as well. If, as a grownup, he finds out that we were not straight with him on certain topics, he might carry over his disappointment with us into other unrelated areas.

We should watch cartoons with our child and not do it as a favor to them. If we do not enjoy this activity, we should let him go to the movies with someone else. When he puts on his Purim outfit, we might want to dress up too. We should cherish all the good moments we spend together. Remember, parents who spend all their time on difficulties and dealing with endless problems are missing out. Such cultural deprivation does not mesh with reality. Children should bring happiness!

The technology of change in children

I meet both parents together only if the friendship between them is solid enough to allow a productive discussion, a kind of staff meeting. If they are at odds with each other and create a negative atmosphere, it is better to meet them separately, or sometimes meet only one of them throughout the process. In our meetings I do not waste time listening to contradictory versions, repetitive complaints or dealing with past, repressed experiences. The focus is on topics that are neglected and repressed at present, while learning a new language of dialogue which is more appropriate for mature abilities.

During my first meetings with parents, I ask each of them to write a page about the other. The page should include a list of abilities, occupations and hobbies. I ask them to be ready to invest in their relationship and go out together more often. I also refer them to texts about raising children.

Meanwhile, they are asked to maintain their relationship with their child as is. Every strategist knows how important it is to keep a secret. If the child notices that the parents are planning something, he might at this early stage, even before the parents have the appropriate tools, challenge them even more and force them to go back to square one. On our second meeting, we go through their lists and choose activities that sound like they would be enjoyable outings. I ask them to go out every night for the next two or three weeks and to plan a weekend for just the two of them. Moreover, we decide what each of them will do separately with the child, and what both of them together will do with him. The activities they choose should be ones that do not trigger the symptom that led them to approach me. If the problem that brought them to me is that the child runs wild a lot, then their activity should take place in an open field.

I explain to the parents that they should promise their child something he has wanted for a long time, without indicating the exact date he will get it. They should think in advance about what it will be, perhaps visiting a water park, getting a new bicycle or a trip abroad? In addition, I tell the parents to hold a short staff meeting every day to coordinate their plans. If, during the day, one of them is not sure about the other's reaction, a telephone conversation is a good idea.

These first meetings are meant to prepare the necessary infrastructure for change. The parents should act as one unit and know their goals and the way to achieve them. Before the change actually occurs, I go over all possible scenarios with them. At first I shoot numerous questions at them and respond to their reactions. If, for instance, the mother says that in a certain situation her child might pretend to be sick so he can stay home and not go to kindergarten, I ask: "So what do you do in a situation like this?" They proffer a few suggestions, while I add some of my own. Only after we have listed some alternative plans for several possible scenarios are they ready to initiate change. This is an important, even critical, week. If they do not manage to produce change, they may reinforce the child's negative behavior. Then, when they try to produce change in the future, they will need more complex strategies.

To increase their chance of success, I back them up throughout the process. During this first week they can call me at any time if something unpredictable happens or just to share some thoughts and experiences with me.

Tonight's entertainment: Bedwetting – A case study

Normally, when growing up, the child wishes to identify with an adult and wants to behave like an adult as soon as possible. But eight-year-old Nathan continued to wet the bed. His parents sent him to a children's therapist. Nathan liked to meet her – she was very nice indeed, and he confided in her. They spoke about fears and anxieties and played different games. Nathan continued to wet the bed even more frequently.

My theory is that Nathan became difficult and clingy just because he was forced to provide his parents with something to deal with. Throughout his early childhood they conveyed the message that in order to keep their attention focused on him intensively, he must arouse their worry and concern.

In fact, bedwetting is a family event. All members of the family take part in it whether they are aware of it or not. The growing child is gradually exposed to reality and has to learn how to deal with its complexity. One of the things toddlers are required to learn is that they should only relieve themselves in a certain place and not anywhere they feel like. This is one of their first encounters with the requirements of reality, and whatever happens in this encounter serves as an infrastructure for social learning as they grow.

If Nathan, a third grader, is still bedwetting, it means he has some kind of developmental delay. It's as if he were asking to sit in a stroller when he already knows how to walk, run and jump. He was demanding that his needs be met immediately while ignoring reality and did not perceive his parents as separate entities. He saw his mother as a supplier rather than a person.

As in many other cases when parents wish to produce change in their children, I suggested that they first invest in their own relationship, and so they did. Soon Nathan noticed that his parents were going out without him. It is important for children to notice that. Eventually they learn not only not to object, but also to wish their parents a pleasant evening.

During the first and second week Nathan said: "Are you going out again? You went out last night!" Parents who want to make changes must be ready to resist all sorts of manipulations that might prevent them from going out. The child might, for instance, cry and complain: "My stomach hurts," or "I am scared to be alone." Obviously, Nathan's parents did not leave him alone, but with a responsible adult. They had to remember that from then on they were not the only answer to his needs and go on with their plans.

When the time came for spending time with Nathan, they used the text they had prepared in advance. His father played football with him and when the game ended, when they were both close and sweaty, he chose to start the conversation with an apology. He said a sentence or two, expressing: "You are not a bad boy, but we, as your parents have been neglectful." Then he added a request: "You are a big boy now, and you shouldn't wet the bed."

"But, dad." Nathan started to say.

Dad knew there was no use discussing the subject, because such discussion once again becomes a family involvement. So he said: "No, I don't want to talk about it. Just remember my request."

Nathan did not stop wetting the bed. So after two or three days, during their time together, the father brought up the subject again. This time he did not use the appeasing, matter-of-fact tone he had used the previous time, but he did not use an angry tone either. "Nathan, have you forgotten what I asked you three days ago?"

"But dad, I can't help it."

Once again the father did not dwell on the subject.

Since there was no change after the second conversation, the parents stopped talking and started doing. Nathan realized his parents were going out more and more without him. They cooperated and treated their son as someone who did not take them seriously and consequently was not worthy of serious consideration. One day Nathan asked his mother about the computer she promised him. The mother was waiting for this question.

"Excuse me," she said, "What are you talking about?"

"The computer, I want."

"Nathan, I will consider your requests the same way you consider mine. Remember what we asked you just a few days ago?"

This is how Nathan learned that he should be considerate towards his parents. He had something to lose.

If Nathan had been older, we could have talked to him more bluntly: "When you decide to grow up, we will talk about it. For now, there is nothing to talk about. Such a gift is not suitable for babies who wet their beds." They could even give him a toy duck to emphasize the point. But such things should only be said by a person who has the appropriate mental budget for them and is able to say it in a totally indifferent tone rather than in a hostile, angry tone.

Nathan's problem was not solved, and his parents moved to the next phase. This time they told him they were going on a weekend with some friends of theirs, but if he continued to wet the bed, they would have to leave him with his grandparents. The child reacted severely and put his parents to the test. He continued to wet as usual, convinced his parents would not be able to go without him. He was wrong. They could and they did. Before going away they had a discussion pretending they did not know he could hear them.

"Where will we leave Nathan for the weekend?"

"At grandma's."

"What will we tell Judy and Mark? How will we explain why Nathan didn't join us?" Judy and Mark were the parents' friends who were going to join them.

"We'll see."

This is how Nathan realized that his parents did not intend to humiliate him by telling the real reason for his absence. This knowledge was extremely important.

Change started after this conversation. Nathan did all he could do in order to be able to join his parents. If, for instance, he had promised his parents that he would change in the future, the parents would have had to go on with their plans and ignore his promises. Such a promise might even bring about a sense of defeat if he tried and did not succeed, and since he was joining his parents anyway and had no reason to try again, he would be left with a sense of failure. On the first days after he decided to make a change, he tried not to fall asleep since he was afraid of wetting the bed while sleeping. His parents were concerned about him, but logic helped them overcome their fears. They knew it was the first step and that eventually Nathan would succeed, just as we grownups, even after drinking a considerable amount of beer, wake up and go to the toilet rather than pee in bed. The parents saw he was trying to change, so they rewarded him by increasing his freedom of movement. They allowed him to join them at various events and on the weekend. He also got a new computer.

After several dry nights, Nathan started bedwetting again. This time his parents pretended not to notice the incident. They knew he was in the midst of the process and did not want to embarrass him. He might wet again from time to time, but eventually he would cease to do it.

When the parents are no longer a couple

When parents are at odds with each other, and I cannot make them cooperate, I meet only one of them. Producing change requires focusing on the able partner rather than on the problematic one, since the able parent is the one who is capable of introducing data which create the dynamics of change. If the able parent is the father, because the mother has already established too complex a relationship with the child, I meet the father separately.

Often the father cannot make his wife spend time with him outside the house. In fact, it is very possible that she is relieved when he goes out by himself. Perhaps she feels more comfortable being alone with her child without her husband. In such cases I search, with the father, for some reasons that will convince her to go out with him. Going out with friends is not recommended, because that will not bring about change. I recommend to the husband to tempt his wife by offering something she really likes, even if he is not particularly interested in it. Perhaps she likes the theater? Or maybe it is worthwhile to subscribe to a series of concerts, lectures or plays? Since payment for these events is arranged in advance, probably the wife would not want to feel that they were wasting their money. Furthermore, I do not reject the option of a more "spiteful" act that might make the wife think twice about her refusal to join her husband – for instance, attending dance sessions with a female friend. If all these methods do not succeed, I tell the father to go out by himself and do it as frequently as possible.

I tell the father: "It's as if you have lost your wife to a lover who happens to be your child." In fact, the father should behave like a divorced man: come home from time to time to take a shower, sleep, eat and spend some time with the child without the wife and let his wife live her own life. The point is that this way, the wife might notice she is becoming a single parent and that her husband is becoming more and more distant. After a while she will probably be willing to cooperate in producing the desirable change. But I am not afraid of saying frankly that if these changes in the father's behavior do not change the mother's attitude within a few months, he should consider a separation. After all, he has already lost his wife, and while living in the house he is not about to derive much pleasure from his child either. It is recommended that he not waste too much time and start planning his own future. Next time around, with a new wife and new children, he will learn from his mistakes and build the new family better from the start.

Nevertheless, it is possible that the mother needs a wake-up call that will encourage her to go beyond the stage she is stuck at. Quite likely, her realization that her husband is about to leave will serve as the wake-up call, and so the husband will eventually stay at home with a new-old child and wife.

If one of the parents has moved forward and established a more diverse and attractive cultural pattern in a new family, the child will react to this parent rather than to the other. It is possible that when the child grows up, he will adjust better to this new family. It is like a child who grows up with parents who speak two languages. In such a case, he speaks both languages fluently, but only one of them is his mother tongue.

***

Childhood is an excellent time for making changes. Most changes in young children are produced easily but need to be thought out. It is more difficult to produce change in older children. In adolescence, change requires more sophisticated methods and the cooperation of the child.

Chapter 12

Change with Adolescents – Busting the Myth

Crisis of adolescence? – Not a must

According to popular myth, our children must go through a serious dilemma, called the "crisis of adolescence." Is this really so?

Parents who reject growth and learning raise their children until they reach a certain predetermined level. Some adolescents who reach this ceiling give up on growing any further and continue to be "good children" in the negative sense of the term. They remain obedient, programmed and limited – as they were brought up to be, without the freedom to explore the world. This situation is not really satisfying for parent or child. Besides, there may be a price to pay later on, when the young person realize it is time to rebel.

Other teenagers continue to develop while staging an awkward revolt against their parents. This option includes multiple obstacles and struggles. Though rebellion has certain advantages, the emotional price it exacts may be a very high one. If the defiance is already evident while the parents keep ignoring the child's striving for independence and maintain an inflexible attitude, the adolescent may feel pushed into a dangerous corner. Parents who limit their teenagers when they are in the midst of change are emotionally static and do not understand the world around them. They are stuck in a place they find comfortable and convinced that the new world their child has entered is defective. This is how huge rifts are created between parents and children.

However, things can be done differently. Using the learning culture, we as parents can enable our teenagers to continue to grow and develop their abilities. Friendly parents benefit from their children's adolescence, a period which enables parents to change the nature of their relationship with their offspring. We should take advantage of the fact that we have more free time and use it to enrich our intimate relationships and our cultural development, while learning a thing or two from our teens. Instead of judging them, we should keep up with them and learn some new things. In this way we will expand our own identity, become familiar with innovations, prepare ourselves for future developments which are bound to happen, get satisfaction from our lives and remain friends with our teenagers.

Instead of rejecting options automatically, it is important that we help our teenagers develop an ability to sort through the various possibilities and choose their own way. Remember that teenagers who are only equipped with crude thinking tools cannot handle the surplus of energies and numerous possibilities they come across. They do not have enough patience to develop their identity and they often need immediate solutions. This is the reason why so many teenagers get confused and caught up in theories which offer a clearly defined identity to people who believe in them. If we equip our children with friendly thinking tools which will help them sort through the numerous stimuli, the years of adolescence may turn into a fascinating period, rich in experiences.

My child's no longer a child

Getting adolescents to change is not that simple. You can yell as loud as you want, dear mom, but your child will probably think you are off the wall. And if dad yells at him, your teenager won't decide that it is time to change his behavior but simply avoid his father.

The source of the distress our children's adolescence may cause us is simple. It seems as if our children were born just yesterday, and we acquired the tools to take care of them, but all of a sudden they are *so* big. Those parents who react with various means of rejection and nag their children constantly tend to lose connection with their children.

Until a short time ago Ron used to love his daughter, to talk to her and hug her frequently. Now that her body has started to develop, he is embarrassed. He does not know where to look and whether it is all right to hug her. Even though the friendship tools Ron used before have become inappropriate, he has not acquired new ones. As a result Ron has become tense, hostile, irritated and aggressive and ready to fly off the handle when his daughter's room is a mess.

Ron's relationship with his son was also simpler in the past, when they used to play together on the lawn. Nowadays they struggle with awkwardness most of the time and do not know how to relate to each other. The son is no longer a child, but neither is he a grownup. What is he?

Because children keep changing all the time, we parents must change with them.

What should we do?

On the whole, we should not tell another person what to do. There are very few situations when people have complete control over others. Examples of such a relationship can be found in prison or in the army, but usually, it is a dangerous illusion to believe that we can control another person. This is particularly true when dealing with teenagers. In most cases when parents treat their adolescents as their subordinates, the teenagers become "offenders." This is how they show off their abilities to people who do not bother to respect them. If we observe our teenagers' abilities with clarity, we will find out that our role as parents has undergone a tremendous change. Teenagers can do whatever they feel like, including things we do not approve of. Teenagers are capable of performing miracles, developing their talents, shaping their identities and enjoying their lives. But they are also capable of foolishness and even of causing disasters.

Consequently, the main question that we, as parents, should ask ourselves is: What can we do which will bring about enjoyment, satisfaction or benefit to ourselves and our teenaged child? The answer to this question is not based on our own past, but rather on our child's future. First, we should check whether we still have something of value to contribute to the adolescent. If the answer is yes, we had better do that. When we act generously we encourage our teenagers to contribute as well. Instead of judging the teenager, we should teach them. If it turns out that our teens still respect us, because of our education, desirable profession or money, and that the teen still loves us and is attached to us, it means we have a common infrastructure which we can use to develop a friendly relationship with him.

But how can we contribute? Suppose, you, the father have studied ancient Greek and you can read Homer. Well done! But if you attempt to pass your knowledge to your adolescent son, you might not act as his friend. Try to think about things that would be relevant for your son at the current time. Perhaps you can study together, for the sake of general knowledge, some challenging subjects such as the human genome? Aside from that, we can turn our son into our teacher, just as if we are using him to expand our world. Many parents find it difficult to understand, just as a few years earlier they found it hard to accept the fact that their ten-year-old son was more adept than them in certain areas. However, that is the way it is. For now, we parents have a slight advantage over our teenagers with regard to finances or other areas they have not yet experienced. But are we as good as they are when it comes to computers? And how about their aptitude for foreign languages? If we decide to be diligent students, there is a chance our teenagers will be patient enough to share their knowledge of electronic gadgets or contemporary music with us, and we will be lucky enough to learn the latest slang. By the way, familiarity with slang is extremely important if we wish to be a part of our adolescents' world.

Once we know our children's world better, we will be surprised to notice how big the generation gap is. It is not only about dress code, but also about social values and agendas. We should adjust to these generational changes. Parents who demand that their teenagers return home by 10 PM make fools of themselves. Many teenagers only start their evening out at midnight, go to bed at dawn and sleep until midday. We too should become more flexible and allow ourselves to do things we have avoided in the past.

If we are not truly learners and find this too burdensome, we should acknowledge this and quit our role as parents. We should step down to allow others to keep on going.

Exercise: Expand your horizons

A teenage girl or boy constitutes a great opportunity for us to expand our horizons, since they can help us to expose ourselves, knowingly, to things we were not exposed to in the past.

So, if the adolescent listens to Eastern music or heavy metal, both of which are alien to us, we should borrow a CD and listen to it. And if our teenage daughter informs us that she has decided to become a vegetarian, and we love meat, we should welcome this opportunity to try some vegetarian dishes.

We have tried. We became familiar with new things. Now, that our horizon is wider, thanks to our adolescent, we can really make a choice.

"Can you say something positive about Mom?"

The language of complaints, which we dealt with in the chapter about spouses, is also a common way of communication between parents and teenagers. We, who find it hard to realize that our children are not kids anymore, may complain about our teenagers' hairstyle, piercings, friends or clothes. Our teenagers, on the other hand, might be exactly at the right age to complain about everything, especially about us – we are fat, boring, know nothing about music and always reject their requests. Often, both parties, parents and adolescents, communicate with each other by using the language of complaints. This language is harmful both to the environment and to the speaker. As parents we must remember that amid endless quarrels, using this language may cause our teenagers to turn a deaf ear to anything we say, even when our criticisms are justified.

Accordingly, if we wish to have a friendly relationship with our teenagers, we must learn how to look at them differently. We should not just keep quiet either. If, for example, we enter our teenage daughter's room and are shocked by the mess but remain quiet, our daughter will read the look on our faces. It is just as if we are again using the language of complaints without uttering a single word. We must avoid this language entirely. We should learn how not to get shocked. There are more important things in life than a messy room. When our teenager complains, we should try first and foremost not to use the same language. Mutual use of the language of complaints leads to an endless battle that worsens by the day. Though we know how it started, we can never know how it will end. If possible, we should answer our teenager with a smile and try to change the subject to a more pleasant one. Besides, it is important not to reject our teenager's claims right away. Later, when we are by ourselves, we should ask ourselves whether there is any truth to them and even try to change accordingly.

Nevertheless, if our teenagers complain endlessly about us, we should not accept all their complaints and try to change. The teenager might start to perceive this language as a positive one since it always produces change. A possible reaction is to create a temporary separation. For example, if our son is hostile and aggressive, and there is no chance of changing the atmosphere, we should change our plans and go to the movies. It will be much more pleasant. If we act this way time and time again, it might bring about change. Our son might learn that when he complains, he does not achieve anything, and he might also lose things he could have had. This method is effective and friendly, at least to us, but on one condition – we must be persistent and determined. We should also remember that the result will not be immediately visible. The language of complaints is difficult to change.

Complaining teenagers find it difficult to see something positive in us. They only see our faults and are almost blind to anything else. Sometimes, when teenagers sit in front of me, I ask them directly: "Can you say something positive about your mom?" Other than that, I give them homework which includes activities that give immediate positive relief, such as sports, music and entertainment.

When the parents are the ones who complain constantly, I might tell them: "I had a really good time with your son. You are supposed to enjoy him even more. I feel sorry for you because you don't. You keep dwelling on the fact that he does not pay enough attention to his studies, but this should be his responsibility. Have you ever noticed his wonderful sense of humor?" Sometimes they blush and then take a positive step on the way to change.

Some things are worse than piercing – Just talk!

As in any other relationship, in order to improve the rapport with our adolescents, we must not fire a series of commands at them.

Instead, we should just talk to them. We should express a personal request. We should offer suggestions they do not want to miss.

What do we usually do? We usually complain about our teenagers' behavior non-stop, and in addition try to convince them to study in a certain high school, choose daddy's profession, wake up early, and avoid being out all night and sleeping all day. We also warn them about cigarettes, drugs and alcohol. Well, this is really silly. We are programmed not to like many things related to youth. We are limited, and each exposure to new things raises negative feelings. Consequently, it is very likely that in most cases we are wrong when we totally reject something our teenager has chosen. But even if we are certain that we are right and think that the teenager must obey us for his own good, it is better not to intervene. In most cases when parents insist on expressing their opinion time and time again, they achieve the exact opposite result. A prohibition might even serve as a trigger to perform the "offence." The adolescents might become even more involved in something we perceive as negative. My own experience has shown that if we are concerned about something but do not manage to conceal our concern from our teenagers, our fears will most probably come true. If we are afraid that our son will become addicted to hard drugs and talk about it nonstop, it will most probably happen. After all, our son is a good kid, and since we are always harping on this subject, he will not disappoint us, and our grim predictions will cause him harm. Only a rebellious teenager will not fulfill our expectations.

In this case particularly, if we wish to give change a chance, we had better choose the most important thing and ignore everything else for the time being. If our greatest fear is the use of hard drugs, our children must realize that crossing this red line will make them lose their place at home. We will not help or support them. We will view drug use as a hostile act which performed against themselves and against us. Such a declaration might well be more convincing than the words of friends who try to convince them to do drugs. But let's make one condition: let's not dwell on the cigarettes, the messy room or the body piercings. Moreover, we might even help our children buy that coveted motorcycle, even though we do not approve of riding them, since a bike may be the lesser of two evils. It is better than hard drugs. Perhaps we might even decide, without telling them, that as long as they only smoke marijuana, we will not say anything, even if it is against the law.

We must not forget that our teenagers are growing up. This is their life, and we cannot assume responsibility for it. In most cases, while we are minding our own business, our teenager will complete the process, will gain experience, will make some mistakes and will become an experienced adult.

Anorexia – A case study

No matter what our teenager's problems are, it is possible and important to encourage a positive change. Such a change might help our teenager to overcome difficulties and depression, assuming that deep down the teenager wants to change but does not acknowledge that.

Molly and Paul, who had an anorexic daughter whom I never met, seemed tired and depressed at our first session. The mother seemed the most miserable and exhausted one because of her daughter's self-destruction. They told me the usual story: a daughter who eats almost nothing, dedicates most of her time to sports to burn off nonexistent fat and vomits out whatever particles of food may enter her mouth.

After listening to their story, I suggested changing the language of communication between the parents and their daughter. I explained that their show of parental concern for their daughter might be harmful for her. The more concern they showed, the faster she deteriorated. I told them that if their daughter was determined to destroy herself, they could not prevent her from doing so. Instead of showing endless concern, I said, the two of them should forget about their role as parents and go out on their own to have a good time. In addition, they were asked to prepare gourmet dinners at home but not invite their daughter to dine with them. They were to explain to her that she could not possibly be good company at such dinners. This was because of her expression of disgust whenever she was forced to eat. I added that there was one particular area where the daughter would be an excellent partner – although they had rejected it so far – sports. Speed-walking would be an excellent pastime for the mother and daughter to share.

"If we do not force her to eat, we will cause more damage!" claimed the mother. "I must at least check what she has eaten and make sure she does not throw up."

"Don't you think you are invading her privacy?"

"But her health."

"Just imagine how you'd feel if your parents insisted on checking your underwear, to see whether you were being hygienic enough, because hygiene is, as you surely know, most important."

The mother was willing to follow my advice. At the end of the session, we agreed that they should not tell their daughter about our sessions. The very thought that her mother and father were consulting with someone might undermine their authority, which was already quite weak in their daughter's eyes.

As a couple Molly and Paul began working on changing the language of communication. They went out every night, left for work early every morning and by doing so managed not to interfere with their daughter's eating habits. When they did find themselves eating dinner with her, they forced themselves to ignore her manipulations. If she joined them at the table without being invited, took only a tiny slice of cheese from the table and then went out in a tracksuit to burn off the calories, the parents continued to mind their own business and play dumb.

The mother chose walking as a shared activity. This was a significant change. Until then they had totally forbidden their daughter to exercise if she did not eat well. The father also pitched in and started bicycle riding with his daughter. All the while, the parents filled the refrigerator with various delicacies, including tasty dishes the mother prepared. They no longer invited their daughter to join them for meals. They started talking in her presence about a trip to France to enjoy gourmet cuisine. The daughter was not included in these plans.

At our third session, the mother said that her daughter did not know how to handle the changes at home. She was confused because she had been suddenly shifted away from the center of family attention to a marginal place. Every once in a while she complained, claiming that her parents did not care about her. The parents continued with their plan, which resulted in an immediate change. Soon the daughter realized she had no audience. No one cared about what she put into her mouth, whether she threw up or not, and whether she exercised or not, so she came to her senses. She worked up an appetite, started to go out in the evenings, and even took tasty food from the refrigerator and ate it. First she did it secretly, when no one was around, and then started to eat in front of others. The family welcomed her back but without any fanfare. In this case, the anorexia turned out to be a passing episode of adolescence, just a brief craziness.

Is there some special formula? Not at all. In a different house, the daughter could have become even more anorexic, in an attempt to make her family react. In cases of such obvious self-destruction, I believe that if teenagers are determined to kill themselves, their parents cannot prevent it. On the contrary, if they try to do so, the situation becomes more dangerous. So, if the struggle to change the language of dialogue does not succeed, the troubled teens should be counseled or hospitalized in facilities where professionals can monitor them.

Sometimes, when it seems that the teenager is determined to remain anorexic, a process which resembles a prolonged suicide, I try to convince the parents to continue to go out together and with the other siblings. Instead of neglecting their daughter's siblings, who witness their parents investing everything they have in the anorexic child, I ask them to invest in those who wish to live. This is not an easy thing to do, but some of those who have followed this advice have managed to do the impossible and promote a change.

No change, no chance

So far I have written what we, the parents, should do in order to form a new relationship with our son or daughter. I have counseled many parents of teenagers, and I am sure that my recommendations help, but they do not solve problems completely. In practice, parents sometimes react to particular provocations by alienating their adolescent even further.

As parents of teenagers we are exposed to an opportunity that we do not necessarily know how to seize. Our children are no longer small, and our own identities have been completely formed. Our financial situation is not bad, and we can really start enjoying life and enjoying each other. Do we do that?

Most parents will give the honest answer that they don't. Many parents even try to reject this opportunity. They are used to working hard and dealing with problems – this is what they do best. This is why they need their adolescents and their time-consuming problems. The teenagers mediate between the parents who have long forgotten what to do in the company of one another. But now, whenever they bump into each other, they discuss one thing, and one thing only – their concerns about their teenager.

The adolescent notices this and does not regard us highly. Consequently, if we wish to influence our son or daughter, we must change. **Really** change. Our teenagers are already familiar with their demanding, irritated parents. They neither respect us nor fear us. We can go on talking until we are blue in the face, but it won't do any good. If we really want to influence our adolescents, we should surprise them by changing contrary to their expectations. They may believe we are weaklings, until all of a sudden mom learns how to ride a motorcycle. If we put enough effort into change, there is a chance our teenager may realize that we can still be of some use and may even try to win our friendship.

The adolescent – Technology of change

First I ask the parents to write a list of all the things they wish to do in the next decade, except for the things they do together with their kids. The list should also include things both parents want to do together to enrich their relationship. I recommend that they renew their relationship and their sex life. They can try new positions in bed. They can go back to school, not to gain academic degrees, but to enjoy themselves. Many parents do not feel like doing any of the above, but sometimes I take advantage of their concern for their child and gain some cooperation. I tell them that as long as they have such limited abilities, their teenagers will continue to disrespect them and their wishes.

If we, the parents, manage to change, and our teenagers continue to ignore us and our wishes and turn the house into a living hell, and such cases do exist, we must use our authority and set limits. We might decide to send the teenager off to a boarding school. Sometimes, when a teenager realizes that parents have lives of their own, they may be inspired to change. If it does not happen, at least we will get our lives back. Our relationship with the teenager does not change, but the daily dictatorship ends.

On the verge of adulthood

Many adolescents do not leave their parents' homes, for economic and other reasons, even after they are no longer adolescents.

However, most teenagers do leave their parents' homes at a certain point and move into a place of their own. Sometimes they move in with roommates, sometimes with spouses and sometimes by themselves. Some of them find it extremely difficult, and as a result they create a conflict with their parents. It is much easier to pick a fight than to say goodbye to your loved ones. In such a case, there is not much we can do at first, besides making the situation even worse. When the adolescents feel safe in their new place and get used to the change, we will reconcile.

A friendly separation has predictable side effects. The adolescent misses his old room. Sometimes he might even shed a tear. Gradually they learn to accept the fact that one stage of their lives has ended and a new one is beginning. At first the teenager will visit the parents frequently, bring his dirty clothes for mother to wash, come by to eat mother's familiar food, and even move back in for a few days when he is sick. All these phenomena and many others are just normal emotional symptoms which will disappear in the course of time.

***

Sometimes, parents go on nurturing their adolescent for a longer period than necessary, not for the teen's benefit, but to solve their own problems. The children have grown up, and the parents have not created new modes of expression for themselves. They know how to take care of children and nothing else. Some children accept the situation readily, glad to remain their parents' kids even after completing their master's degree. On the whole, everybody suffers from this situation: the thirty-year-old children who fail to make a life for themselves and the parents who do not take advantage of the wonderful gift they have received, which is called free time.

Chapter 13

Never Stop Changing

A new phase has begun

The changes we undergo are not only related to our career, our spouses and our children; they occur throughout life. Children leave the nest and start families of their own. Our parents, who once were strong and supportive, need care themselves. We become grandparents. Our health is not what it used to be.

As we age, we have fewer resources and less energy. Change becomes a bigger challenge and requires strict prioritization before we decide where to invest our limited strength and time. We pay a higher price for our mistakes, since we have less time to fix them and to learn lessons from them, to start something from scratch and to succeed. We also have more to lose.

I do not wish to define the word "mistake." If, for instance, one spouse wants to get a divorce, the future may reveal that this decision was a mistake, and there will be a price to pay. But the decision to stay with his wife and get old together might turn out to be wrong as well. The question of correct and incorrect cannot be answered by using a certain formula. However, at a mature stage in our lives, we must dedicate more time to friendly thinking, to planning and making decisions before acting.

Moreover, it is important that we do not stop learning until our final day. We should meet people whose experience and abilities can enrich us. Likewise, when we have something to contribute, we should teach others, which will help us improve our own abilities. We can also take up new hobbies, visit new places and so on.

During the second half of our lives, we should persist with the friendly principle of developing existing abilities and not suffer from the lack or decline of other abilities. If we concentrate on our diminishing abilities, we will find ourselves in the shoes of the woman who bases her identity on her looks and now suffers from the fact that she is aging. So, we should continue to play tennis, but we might want to change our style a little. We should stop dancing hip-hop and throwing ourselves on the floor, but we might want to take up ballroom dancing or folk dancing. Some abilities improve with time. Let's focus on them.

When children leave the nest

We have been parents for many years, and all of a sudden our home is empty. Now it seems bigger and quieter. How do we experience this drastic change? Our grownup children no longer give us a chance to express ourselves. They have become parents and are increasingly less dependent on us. In many fields they are more talented than we are. Consequently we are left with a need to give which we cannot fulfill. This is the time to change our relationship with our children, to talk with them as adults, to listen to their advice about subjects we used to advise them about not so long ago. True, they still ask our opinion every now and then, but it comes from a different place, since they know that senior wisdom is valuable. However, family relationships, as good as they might be, no longer require the great energies we invested in the past. As a result, we are left with time and energy we need to invest elsewhere.

People whose whole identity is based on raising young children might find themselves in a crisis. Some start taking care of their old parents as a full time job. Those whose identity is not based on taking care of others maintain a steady, good relationship with their parents but use alternative solutions, such as hired help, when it comes to their daily care. They too might find out that their time and resources are not used to a full extent.

Unfortunately, the void that is created after older children leave is sometimes filled up with illness, problems with the younger children, quarrels, suffering and even financial problems. We are supposed to be wealthier now, moving on to the next phase of life and enjoying comfortable living, but sometimes we do not seize this wonderful opportunity.

Linda (46) worked as a bookkeeper in a bank. She got married at a young age and soon became a mother. Recently both her children moved out of the house. At the bank, the young employee who sat next to her told her about his life from time to time. He had a girlfriend, and they were planning a long trip abroad. Linda fell in love with this young man. She started dreaming about him at night and looked forward to meeting him in the morning. She knew he did not even notice her as a woman. For him she was an older friend, perhaps even a mother figure. She saw him as an attractive man. The fact that she had no chance of ever fulfilling her dreams brought on depression. She faced a dead-end. Although the young man excited her, she stood no chance. He would never be her lover or her partner.

Her relationship with her husband was very limited and quite dull. She had never taken a lover, and it was pointless to tell her to find one. Because she was very stimulated and could not find any direct relief, I recommended channeling this stimulation to a place where she could express herself - to her relationship with her husband. Her imagination was not a friendly place and had robbed her of valuable energies. Linda initiated some changes in the bedroom which her husband accepted gladly. In addition, she initiated some social and cultural outings and went places with her grownup children. Soon she started to feel better about herself, her husband and her children. When her male colleague flew abroad, she said goodbye affectionately without much regret.

Linda had other possibilities to choose from. She could have learned a new profession, like a teacher I know who retired and started a second career marketing textbooks. Acquiring a new ability such as embroidery or a foreign language could also have improved her self-esteem and confidence.

Surprisingly, at this stage of our lives, we have numerous possibilities to choose from. One particularly friendly opportunity is the connection between grandparents and grandchildren. Grandchildren give us the chance to spend some quality time with our families. The grandchildren meet grownups who are often willing to devote a great deal of time to them, much more than their busy parents can provide. Grandparents are able to spend much more time with their grandchildren than they could with their own children. Our children also benefit from the deal. Assuming that family relationships are normal, most of them would rather leave their children with their parents than with a babysitter or a nanny. Developing such a relationship is highly recommended and benefits all family members.

Grandchildren as peacemakers – A case study

In cases where family relationships have soured, grandchildren can sometimes bridge the gaps between parents and their grown children. This is what happened when Rebecca and Albert became parents. Rebecca, the apple of her parents' eyes, was born in Israel but was raised in accordance with European culture. When she started dating Albert, whose family came from North Africa, her parents were totally shaken. It did not match the various scenarios they had in mind for their daughter. They attacked the relationship savagely to no avail. On the contrary, their attacks only strengthened the young couple's relationship. Albert's family also reacted with surprise, but in a milder, teasing way. They kept saying that Albert had fallen for someone who would never be perfect for him, meaning that Rebecca would never learn how to cook the family favorites, even if she tried really hard.

Rebecca told Albert about her parents' fierce objections, even providing some exact quotes. She should not have done that in my opinion, since insults are not easily forgiven. Albert, whose feelings were hurt, told Rebecca he would never enter her parents' house and made it clear he would not welcome her parents into his house either. Moreover, he gave Rebecca an ultimatum to choose between him and her parents. He added that if she met up with them, he would see it as a betrayal.

Rebecca stopped seeing her parents, and the situation remained unchanged for a long time. Meanwhile she adjusted well to Albert's large family, where she found warm, affectionate people who liked to hug, sing and laugh. She had a new family that was perhaps too daunting at times. Although the couple did not have a subscription to the philharmonic, Rebecca didn't find that to be a serious problem. Once in a while she talked on the phone with her mother in secret, but because her mom complained so much about the distress Rebecca was causing them, their talks became even less frequent.

Before the wedding all parties involved felt they might have gone too far, and that it was time to make peace. However, soon the hesitant negotiations between Albert's uncle and the bride's brother-in-law ran aground. Rebecca's parents were afraid that Albert's family was after their money, then a new argument broke out about the choice of rabbi to officiate at the wedding, and the negotiations came to a dead end. Rebecca's parents were not present at the wedding.

A year later a baby was born, and when he turned two, Rebecca's parents came to see me. Their complaint was that they had only wanted the best for their daughter, and couldn't understand why they were getting punished for that. The grandson clinched matters for them. They were eager to see him and did not know what to do.

I did not agree with their interpretation of the situation. Instead, I suggested they view the situation as a cultural misunderstanding, very common among new immigrants. Though Rebecca's parents had lived in Israel for decades, I intentionally used the term "new immigrants." I perceived them as such because their point of view had remained the same. They had simply not adjusted to the culture of the new country. Then I offered them two alternatives. The first one was to leave the situation as is and be willing to pay the price – an unbridgeable gap between them and their daughter and grandson. The second alternative was to invest in some cultural learning and then venture a peacemaking attempt which might actually work this time. I assume that if the grandson had not been born, they would have remained in their cultural isolation, but eventually they chose the second alternative.

So they could get to know Albert and his family's culture, they were asked to do several things: listen to Eastern music, eat out a number of times in Eastern restaurants and read several books. Then they were to call Rebecca, telling her that they had met me, that I had criticized them for their behavior, and that I requested one meeting with her. I felt that after hearing of my criticism, she would agree to come and not be afraid it was just another attempt to win her over to her parents' views.

Rebecca came and even agreed to cooperate, acting as a cultural mediator between the two families. At first she talked to Albert's mother and told her about her parents. Then she talked to her parents and described her new relatives. Later Rebecca's parents asked to meet with Albert's mother. A friendship began to form, tentative at first but positive. Rebecca's parents got to know an interesting family and gorgeous grandson, while the child gained another set of grandparents. Finally Albert even agreed to taste some new dishes which his mother had not prepared.

Doctor, I'm sick – Psychosomatic diseases

Sometimes, when we have too much free time, we find a new pastime, which in the past we did not have enough time and energy for – illnesses. This preoccupation is like any other pastime. In fact, it might be even more addictive. Contrary to common assumptions, I believe it is much easier to suffer than to enjoy oneself. In order to learn to enjoy ourselves, a special learning effort is needed, whereas indulging in pain and suffering (or inflicting pain and suffering on others) is freely available. Spending time on medical examinations and various treatments is easy. In my opinion, those of us who wish to view themselves as healthy people must decide they are part of the learning culture. After joining this culture, we can sometimes overcome pain. We can decide to spend time on some intense activity which will make us forget about the pain, or at least make it bearable. Sometimes when people claim it is hard for them to concentrate for long periods of time because of pain, I disagree with them. They are obviously able to concentrate on the pain quite impressively. If they use this magnificent ability and learn how to concentrate on music, on other people and on interesting activities, they will have an opportunity to shape their days according to something which is unrelated to pain or disease.

We should realize that people who feel bad and consider themselves unhealthy as a result are likely to become sick. Stomach aches will turn into an ulcer; arrhythmia will become heart disease. Just as playing the piano all day long will turn a person into a pianist, so one who spends all his time on medical issues will develop the identity of a sick person. Millions around the world take their body temperature every day, even several times a day. How important is it to know your exact body temperature? In cases when this information is really essential, our body will tell us immediately, even without a thermometer. Are the slight changes really that significant? The same question can also be asked about people who check their blood pressure several times a day.

Joey suffered severe chest pains. I was under the impression that it was psychosomatic. Just to be on the safe side, I suggested he undergo some medical tests, but no pathological evidence was found. I assumed the pains were related to anxiety, and the timing reinforced my assumption. Joey had just quit his job to launch his own business, and his previous employer would now become one of his clients. This was a significant advance and a drastic change. Joey's homework included energetic athletic activities, livening up his relationship with his wife and spending time with his grown children, besides promoting the success of his new office.

When we met a week later, Joey chose to talk about his business and about his relationship with his wife and children. He did not even mention his health condition. He managed to improve his private and professional life and stopped seeing me after four sessions. Nowadays I read about him in the financial media from time to time and enjoy reading about his success.

Obviously, as we become older, we experience various diseases and pains. Backaches, for example, might be frequent. However, some people choose to shape their identity according to these illnesses, while others don't. Pain does not force us to take on the identity of a sick or a handicapped person. We can keep our identity as a musician, a singer, an economist, a family man, an intellectual, and so on. We should integrate our limitations into the other components of our identity. Sometimes the physical limitation of one person is no different from the limitation of another who is not defined as handicapped. The limitation of the latter is not physical but is reflected in other areas, such as an inability to be empathic to other people.

I cannot resist the temptation to add a few words about the doctors in whom we trust. I see many of them (though not all), just as I see many psychologists and educators (again, not all) as nothing more than secretaries. The doctor-secretaries compartmentalize people according to a diagnosis and treat them according to this classification. Secretaries who know how to file documents well might be needed in an office. However, this way of acting is totally scandalous when dealing with people who, out of pure ignorance, consent to bureaucracy and spend all their time in medical facilities.

The doctor-secretaries have a computer and forms with various test results printed on them, and treat the patient without really knowing the person, touching his body or giving him any specific attention. These doctors' sole concern is for themselves – they want to cover themselves and avoid litigation. They do not think creatively, nor are they friendly to the patient. We must remember that we are dealing with our lives, and must not trust these secretaries with our lives. Ultimately we should be the ones who decide what is best for us.

In principle I do not oppose the use of medication. Friendly thinking, which includes the search for friendly paths and creating friendly scenarios, takes whatever is worthwhile from analytic thinking, just as it does not rule out magical thinking. However, I prefer to promote the concept of personal ability as much as possible, in health issues as in any other area. It would be much better to reduce our blood pressure by regular physical activity, a friendly diet or biofeedback, through which a person controls the processes that take place in his body. However, if all of the above do not suffice, of course we should take medication that regulates our blood pressure so that we can live a normal life.

Death around the corner – A terminal disease?

We cannot ignore the fact that eventually our health does deteriorate, and diseases progress until the point where death appears on the horizon. I have accompanied some terminal patients until the end.

Medicine has developed tremendously throughout the years and can cure many diseases that were untreatable in the past. Various operations, chemotherapy and other means can cure cancer. However, there is a stage at which medicine can no longer help. Some patients continue to undergo harsh treatments and suffer from their side-effects until the day they die, passing away in great agony. Some people prefer to pray, others consult with mystics.

Dealing with the angel of death is very complex. Can one befriend death? Can one choose a friendly death? I think it is possible. I also believe it is important to do so since knowing death can improve our lives.

Hannah went to the hospital for a simple, trivial examination. She found out she had aggressive cancer which had metastasized all over her body. When the doctors suggested radiotherapy and chemotherapy, Hannah refused and chose alternative medicine. When she came to see me she truly believed she would beat the disease. She told me enthusiastically about Reiki treatments and various foods and beverages that were prepared especially for her. She meditated a lot and did all sorts of things I am not familiar with. I thought she looked worse every time she came to see me, but since she said she felt so good, I kept quiet and hoped she would continue to feel this way. In this case, faith did not save her life. She passed away within a few months, but she managed to avoid suffering and to enjoy her existence. Every now and then we hear about patients whose faith can lead to remission.

Jerry found another solution for his approaching death. When he became ill with cancer he was rather young. He loved extreme sports and seemed the last person who was likely to become ill. Since he was not used to associating with doctors and healers, he ignored all the early signs and went to the doctor when it was already too late. When the doctors suggested chemotherapy, he refused just like Hannah. In fact, he was the client who taught me about the option we have not to put our lives in the hands of "medical secretaries" who tend to experiment and rob us of our right to end our lives with dignity.

At our first session I asked him whether he knew he was about to die. Contrary to so many others, who behave as if they are unaware, Jerry said he knew. Then I asked him what he would like to do in the remaining time and suggested he make a list of ideas. The result was overwhelming. It was as if he had immediately turned into a philosopher. He established a sharp distinction between things that were important and things that were insignificant. His priorities became crystal clear to him. First, he asked the doctors to reassure him that he would not suffer too much pain. Secondly, he wanted to take care of all matters and leave his wife and children a clean slate, so he wrote a detailed will. Then he prepared a personal list of all the things he wished to do before the end came. The list itself is not that important since it reflected his personal preferences, but I will mention some of its items. Though he had always wanted to go to New Zealand, he decided that nothing would happen if he did not go there. Instead, he wanted to write a book before he died. And so he did. Someone else might have fulfilled a particular fantasy, such as having sex with an Asian woman or spending a huge amount of money on a work of art. Another might choose to reread the books he had read during his adolescence, while yet another one would rather study mysticism. Jerry lived for another year, which he claimed was the best year of his life, and I believed him.

I also met people who were busy with numerous activities meant to prolong their lives. They are still with us. Perhaps some of the changes they made after they had found out they were sick led to their recuperation.

Task: Order of priorities

It is important that we define for ourselves the path to follow throughout our lives. The path to follow in the second part of our lives is less clear than that of the earlier years. At that point, many people choose to build a family and a career. To decide which direction to follow, we must ask ourselves an important question: if we had only three months to live, what would we do with the time? Although this question is relevant to people of all ages, there is a better chance that an older person will take it seriously and answer it sincerely. The answers might clarify matters for us, help us organize our priorities and take action.

Remember, **we will all die** eventually. It is better not to ignore this fact and not to waste our time and energy on nonsense.

Friendly accompaniment

This section of the book describes the friendly counseling I provide for clients, sometimes for couples, and is described primarily from my viewpoint.

I call the first sessions "brain meetings" because intensive learning takes place there. I study the people in front of me and their situations, while my clients learn the language of friendly thinking. Together we build the working tools which will enable people to change their identities. We define the language we will use and examine the abilities that should be promoted. To achieve maximal impact, we meet as frequently as possible at this stage. When the clients are ordinary, normal people, only three brain meetings are needed.

Then come the "work meetings," during which I accompany the changes. My aim is to make this process as effective and short as possible. These sessions are extremely practical. We go through the homework the client has done and decide on future homework. The number of these sessions and their frequency varies, but most of the time we only have a few sessions.

Besides describing our sessions from my point of view, I will include some of my clients' accounts. Here I asked them to describe the meetings a long time after they had occurred and permanent change had set in. This peek into my office is not intended to reveal any magic formula relating to my friendly accompaniment. Another friendly coach might develop different methods. However, one thing should be common to us all – the process of change.

Chapter 14

The First Meeting is the Most Important

What's it all about? I gather information

The first meeting, in which I try to gather as much information as possible, might last for an hour-and-a-half or even two hours. When I abandoned clinical psychology, I also changed the conventional time limit for therapeutic sessions. If people make the effort to come to see me, despite traffic jams and parking issues, I adjust my schedule and offer them all the time they need.

I normally start with the question: what brings you here? Usually the answer is a complaint about something. I listen to the client for a few minutes and let him choose the topic. I listen to his message and his way of thinking. I listen to the way he chooses to talk, the way he selects words. While the client is talking, I complete my initial review: I concentrate on the message this person sends, on what his eyes convey. If a couple is involved, I can see at this early stage whether they are friends or not. Sometimes I can even sense that the wife has stopped loving her husband or that the husband is depressed.

I do not look for this type of information actively. It is just there for me to see or sense. Those who deal with people all the time, regardless of their exact profession, sense various things about their clientele even before they start speaking. I learn a lot from the data they provide, although they do not intend to reveal some of it even to themselves.

Susan (35) was quite an attractive woman who did not seem to be depressed or suffering. She was single and had been feeling quite lonely recently. She still lived with her parents. Her mother was a teacher and her father a salesman. She had six sisters and was the third child in the family. All of her sisters, including the younger ones, were married, and three of them lived abroad. Although she was the graduate of a teachers' college, she worked as a secretary in an insurance company. Previously she had worked as a secretary in a law firm. She rarely went out after working hours. She had not had a romantic relationship with a man for quite a long time and had never lived with one. She'd had several incomplete relationships, the longest of which lasted for three months.

She provided all this information in the first five minutes of our meeting. What did I learn from these facts? I learned that Susan was still single – not because there were not enough men in the world, and not because men never approached her – but because she had actively dismissed them until now. In addition, I understood that what defined her was a failure to progress, and not only regarding her relationships with men. Where work was concerned, she worked in temporary jobs and avoided the teaching profession she had trained for, the same profession her mother had practiced for many years. In short, Susan refused to grow and succeed. Some kind of obstacle was preventing her development.

I hypothesized that perhaps her sisters had managed to start families and shape professional identities because they'd moved abroad – far away from the influence of their parents. Perhaps Susan remained so close to her parents at the expense of investing in her personal development. It was as if she was not allowed to achieve in areas where success could not be hidden, such as work and marriage. I put this assumption at the back of my mind and continued to survey what was in front of my eyes with all its endless shades and complexities. I always make sure not to stick to a single conclusion and to remain open-minded.

During our conversation, Susan agreed to accept my assumption about the similarities between her professional and private lives. She said she was willing to change dramatically and expand her range of motion. She understood that she had a choice to make. She could try entertaining men and developing herself while remaining in her parents' home, or she could move out of their house and live independently. She was even willing to consider teaching, an occupation she had regarded as her mother's exclusive domain. It was not complicated. It was all about not waiting for change to occur, but to become active, arbitrarily at first. Soon she might find herself enjoying the process. If she did not start acting independently, she would probably remain stuck in place.

At the first meeting, however, I cannot yet predict the client's learning ability. If I diagnose each client according to the way he sounds at this stage, the results will not be flattering. This is because at the first meeting, most clients seem awkward and set in their ways. I force myself to wait a little and see what the future holds. During the next sessions clients start the process of change and soon they feel and speak differently.

The guy in front of me is broken-hearted. His partner recently left him and moved out. He seems a total wreck, has not slept for some nights and does not even go to work. He is not crazy and is willing to talk about the situation soberly. He claims that he understands what has happened and is even willing to assume some of the responsibility. His topics of conversation are limited in the extreme – she. she. and she. His point of view is so limited that I feel he is almost blinded. His whole being is focused on the return of his loved one.

He suffers a storm of emotions, during which tears stream down his cheeks. I only wait a moment. I must distinguish between crying as a habit or a language, and crying as a reaction to a traumatic event. Obviously, if I come across a person who has just experienced a disaster, I can only offer my condolences. It is not the right time for psychological therapy or learning of any kind, and it is better to postpone the meeting. But when we are dealing with an event that has taken place several months earlier or a problem which has existed for a long time, I feel that the client is crying in my presence because he has gotten used to crying.

Sometimes I offer the crying client some friendly first aid and suggest that he devote two or three days to intensive athletic activity such as walking long distances or possibly running. Sports will bring him some positive relief that will enable him to graduate to more productive activities. Several days of intensive athletic activity generally improves the situation. However, if the client cannot force himself into this regime, or if he does but fails to emerge from his depression, I send him to a psychiatrist who will prescribe medication. This medication is not a permanent solution but will bring about a rapid upturn that will enable the production of more effective solutions. Wallowing in suffering is not beneficial, and a person must do whatever he can to minimize it.

During this specific meeting I felt I was dealing with habitual crying, which I tried to stop immediately. I did not sympathize with the client, but instead posed some matter-of-fact questions that eventually forced him to wipe his eyes and answer me. Since we were dealing with a specific event, I asked him to tell me exactly what happened. He wiped his eyes and started talking: "She's a parasite. I picked her up from the street and gave her a home and attention. She's ungrateful. I only told her she was wrong to make me wait without being in touch. Obviously I was upset and yelled at her, because it wasn't the first time she'd done such a thing, but she didn't understand. Instead of saying she was sorry, she told me to stop yelling at her. Then she slammed the door and went out. She came back later, not because she wanted to talk or apologize, but just to pack some things and leave." He felt terrible and was sure she had found someone else to live with.

I immediately noticed that he, like most clients at a first meeting, was presenting a mixture of information, judgments, opinions and diagnosis. He perceived his own opinions as clear, reliable facts and not as mere assumptions. I interrupted him, explaining that he should think of me as a student who wished to learn his personal language. What did he mean by the word "parasite"?

He explained that she had not worked lately. In the past, she had worked in an office for a year-and-a-half and left when a former employee returned. I kept asking him to translate the terms he used and got the following picture from his answers: this was not the first time that such an event had taken place, following a particular pattern. She would do something he considered wrong, he would criticize her and preach at her, then she would counter attack. Next he would get angry and raise his voice, until everything blew up and they stopped speaking to each other. After these quarrels, they would become quiet and avoid each other. A few days or weeks late, their fury would subside and they'd make peace, mostly in bed, until next time. The fact that the couple had developed this clear, well-defined language of communication made him complacent. Although he was certain they would always stay together, this time she surprised him. She chose a new reaction and walked away. He felt as if the whole structure he'd created had collapsed.

I concluded that the person in front of me was not a good learner, since he followed, time and time again, a pattern which always led to a quarrel. Now I thought it was time to end this part of the session. He had talked about himself more than enough.

As you see from my descriptions of these sessions, my method differs from that of canonical psychology, in which the therapist tries to talk as little as possible and leaves the floor to the patient. I listen to first-time clients only for a few minutes, primarily to grasp the language of their thinking. Then I interrupt them and start creating the tools for friendly thinking. This is not easy for some people, especially if they have already experienced psychological therapy. They wish to talk without interruption. I believe that if the same old pattern of client monologue and passive listening by the therapist will define our sessions too, the client will continue to live with the same tools he has been using. In this case, the client will not change but only "recycle" himself. That is why I don't perceive the listening, especially at the first meeting, as a friendly act. At a later stage, I will listen to the client if he does his homework and sharpens his thinking tools.

However, sometimes I let clients speak about themselves when they are overwhelmed by emotions. There are also first sessions, in which

I allow my clients to deviate from the purpose of the meeting and indulge in small talk that includes jokes, discussing movies and so on. I do not wish to be harsh and inflexible. But I make one condition: the client must be aware that we are exchanging pleasantries and chatting, not focusing directly on core matters. I believe that chatting too can serve a purpose, even discussing things that seem irrelevant. I am not sure one can know for certain what is relevant and what is irrelevant right at the beginning.

Nevertheless, in most meetings, at this point I open a file, grab a pencil and start asking questions prepared in advance. If the client has a spouse or a longtime boyfriend or girlfriend, I ask about them first. I asked the young man described above about the woman who had left him: What's her name? How old is she? What does she do? He was surprised: Why wasn't I asking about him? Why her? I deliberately didn't answer this question because I wanted to save him from himself and force him to refer to someone else or something else. This is how I start the learning activity from the very first session. A learning activity means going beyond our narrow limits so we can then focus on someone else or something else. If a client has children, I ask him about them. If he is a divorced man, I ask him to tell me a little about his former wife. How long were they together? How long have they been divorced? I talk about his partner. How many siblings does she have? I write down their occupations and whether or not they are married. I also write down their husband's occupation.

Here too, when people answer questions about others, some express opinions about the other people in the belief that they are stating objective facts. This is how another client of mine, a married man, reacted when I asked him what his wife does: "She doesn't do anything."

He probably meant she did not work outside the house, not considering her household chores as work. I immediately reacted: "I didn't ask you to express your **opinion**, I asked you to tell me what she does."

He came to his senses and started providing information. "She takes care of the house and the children, cleans, does the laundry, cooks." Now it sounded more accurate.

"And the child?" I ask another client, "What does he do?" She also believes she is answering my question and does not notice that she is providing information about the things her child doesn't do: "He is not a good student, he refuses to go to school, he doesn't obey his parents."

I interrupt her and ask her to describe what the child actually **does** – plays football, plays computer games, watches TV. At this point I do not accept any judgments without reacting. I consider keeping quiet to be an unfriendly reaction since it abandons clients to their ignorance. I try to use an amused tone so as not to hurt their feelings.

For example, when a woman client tells me the man she is interested in makes her suffer, and often claims he does not have time to meet her, I ask her: "Why do you want him so badly?"

She says: "Because he is gorgeous, attractive and interesting."

She still does not know that these words only reflect her own feelings. I can act surprised and say, "Are you telling me you have found the only real man in the Middle East, and that's why you are so attached to him?"

After a smile crosses her face, we can then move forward. She will start to realize that she has decided that this man will be a big part of her life, even though he does not have a developed friendly ability or has not chosen her as a girlfriend, and that she is interested in him for the wrong reasons.

Perhaps the fact that I interrupt my clients after a naïve sentence gives the impression that I am nitpicking. But this session, dedicated to learning the language of thinking, involves changing our previous lexicon of thought. That is why I seize every opportunity to teach my client our new language. Since most people confuse facts with interpretations, I try to promote the language of facts as the one we are about to use in our sessions. Likewise, I aim to differentiate between objective facts, on the one hand, and diagnosis and interpretations, on the other.

Following a brief gathering of data related to the partner in question, I go back to the client. I write down his name, ask him his age, his occupation, and how long he has been practicing it. If it is a rather new occupation, I might ask him about his previous employment. Then I ask him how long he has been with his partner. At this point I cannot possibly know which questions are relevant, so I continue to gather information and ask further about the occupations of his parents and his partner's parents. I try to understand his background as much possible and perhaps even get some hints regarding his direction in life. If, for instance, he is an educated person who comes from an uneducated family, perhaps the fact that he did not follow in his parents' footsteps is an indication of an amazing ability which can be tapped to produce future change.

I continue to use the language of facts and do not hesitate to interrupt the client when he utters a sentence he views as informative and I view as judgmental.

"I am very comfortable at my parents' house," says 30-year-old Guy, who is unemployed, a virgin, and has never lived anywhere else. I say that he might feel at ease now because he can't compare it to anything else. He is inexperienced, and his parents' house is the only place he is familiar with. Once he starts a process of growth and development he will discover many pleasant, comfortable, fascinating and rewarding places. I make sure he has heard this, and only then do I resume listening.

First I try to find out about the areas in which he has ability. Then I ask him to use the tools available to him in these areas and apply them to other, weaker areas. We have already prepared the infrastructure for a language of friendly dialogue in areas which serve the main interest of this particular individual.

Preparing for the next meeting

It's time for homework now.

I tell the client that I do not have enough details yet, so the homework will help me collect the missing information. Many people do not like homework, especially not the kind that needs to be written down. I explain that the tasks are for their own good, not mine. We need the homework in order to move on. It is meant to shorten the process. Without homework, we will need many meetings just for the purpose of gathering information, and it will require much more time and money.

Besides, I tell my clients I am not about to focus on the object of their complaint. If a client complains about his wife, the complaint only testifies to his ability, not hers. If parents complain about their children, I see the children as perfectly normal, and the parents or the language of the house as factors that require change. I ask my clients to write down their homework and to do a little reading. The reading includes material I have written in the past about the matter in question. The written homework, at this stage, includes preparing several lists.

The first list includes everything the clients do these days and everything they have ever done. I ask them to include the things they actually **do,** rather than the things they **do not do**. The list should be very detailed and not be written in a certain order, but according to associations, and most important, all opinions and judgments must be left out. It should include everything from preparing eggplant salad through swimming to salsa dancing. If the client once rode a bicycle or played the flute, but does not do it anymore, I ask him to indicate it as a past activity. This is the most important list since it constitutes an infrastructure for the future work plan.

The purpose of the second list is to provide information about the people who are part of my client's everyday life: spouse or partner, children, parents (if the client still lives with them) business partner, roommate. Usually I focus on the individual the client perceives as the source of the problem. For example, I ask the client to write down information about his wife – the things he knows she does nowadays, the things she has done in the past. I ask him to write about the things she likes to do while watching her favorite TV show – eating popcorn or having her spouse kiss her ears. I do not intend to pry. My purpose is to check how well my client knows his spouse. I repeat that I am not asking for opinions of any kind. All I request is factual data.

The third list includes all the activities my client and the other person have done together or still do together. If my client is a single person who is looking for a mate, like Susan, I ask them whether he or she has had a long relationship in the past, and then ask for a report about this former partner and about the things they used to do together.

Sometimes the homework includes more than just the lists. It might include a significant action. I suggest that the young man that still lives with his parents and has never supported himself should earn a few bucks so he can start creating a professional identity. It would not bother me if he delivered newspapers or worked in a gas station. To my client, the young man I described before that was dumped by his girlfriend, I say, "If I were a wizard, I would have made you fall in love with another woman. Since I'm no wizard, I am willing to compromise. If you are willing to spend a few nights in the bed of a female friend, even one you aren't attracted to, you will do yourself a favor. You will suffer less, and it might change something for the woman who decided to leave you. Ask someone to be your babysitter because you are afraid to sleep alone."

I offered this man a piece of advice, but was aware that he had not yet acquired the friendly tools to use it. So, what was it worth? Perhaps he would learn that it is preferable not to spend the next few nights on his own, that he had better find another solution. If, by any chance, he managed to surprise us both by taking my advice, he would immediately feel better and we could move forward.

However, since in this particular case, we did not know for sure that his girlfriend had left for good, and it was definitely possible they would get back together, I offered another piece of advice. If she gave him a chance, he should grab it at once, but he must change the pattern they had created together. This time, instead of criticizing and attacking, he should remain friendly and look for more effective responses.

I do not set a date for our second meeting because I want to avoid the mind-numbing routine that is typical of psychological therapy, when people meet in the same place at the same time for years. Some clients insist on making an appointment so that they can feel committed. Although I agree, I emphasize that we will not be able to move forward without the written task.

As for the course of development, I emphasize from the start to my clients that unless they are willing to learn a new method, we will not be able to proceed. My clients must be learners. I further stress that I do not expect them to entertain me indefinitely with details of their crises or to support me financially. My guiding principle is for them to derive benefit and make changes in their lives as quickly as possible so they do not need me anymore.

If you have not internalized the fact that I offer a process of learning rather than psychological therapy, I must explain that the meetings are no different from any other learning session. We can decide to learn typing or computer software by ourselves, using books and practice, or through a structured course.

The first meeting in the client's eyes

Many of my clients considered the first session a difficult one. Many told me, after a while, that they did not understand anything during the first session and sometimes even during the second one. So why did they keep coming? Most of them told me that they came after they met an acquaintance who had changed tremendously. He prepared them by telling them the beginning would be difficult but promised that, if they were persistent, they would be able to achieve their goals.

I try to simplify my words as much as I can, but sometimes my clients don't understand the new way of thinking I'm suggesting. Their thinking tools were created many years earlier, and they are usually fixated on analytic-logical and psycho-logistic thinking. They find it hard to change their operating systems. It is quite possible that when I talk about the need to create a unified language for me and the client, I actually talk in a language of my own, and the clients do not understand a thing.

From clients' reactions I learned that sometimes, the first sessions provide a shock similar to that which an immigrant experiences in a new country. If I were to adjust myself to the person in front of me, it would be easier for them to adjust as well. But I believe that if I were to accommodate myself to my clients, they would remain stuck in their own world. That is why I remain faithful to my method, and the client must make an effort to learn the language of friendly thinking. By the way, I also believe this is true for new immigrants. Those who expect the new country to conform itself to the culture they came from remain stuck in a cultural ghetto, and the ones who gradually learn the new culture will eventually adapt.

Another reason for the shock some clients experience at our first meeting is my extreme enthusiasm about this chance, perhaps the only chance, to penetrate the armor they have created and lay the groundwork for friendly thinking. If I don't manage to do it now, I might not get another opportunity. I feel an affinity with the sperm frantically racing to fertilize an egg. Though I am aware that my enthusiasm might alienate some clients, and I may be overdoing things, I simply can't help it.

Unlike people who do not understand my language, others gradually redden in the face from impatience. They have understood me from the start and wish to move on. However I keep giving them examples as if I don't appreciate their intelligence. Because I am not sure that they understand, I continue explaining.

Unfortunately, some first meetings are doomed to failure. During the session I explain the term inept rejection, but if a client is rejecting me, they end up without the tools with which they can progress. Despite what I say about the thinking process, all they hear is the bottom line. They are convinced that I have strong opinions that clash with their own strong opinions, so they reject everything I say as unfounded. Such clients may even start an exhausting argument that leads nowhere. In such a case, there is no point in meeting again. I wish I were not tempted to be dragged into controversies. This is a mistake on my part, as the client only becomes more convinced that I am an arrogant person who thinks everybody else is a fool, and gets very irritated with me.

Danny, who was once a confirmed bachelor, and is now a married man and a father, told me that during the first meetings he tried really hard to restrain himself and not react, even though he did not agree with me at all.

"I was sitting in front of a person who spoke nonsense."

So why did he continue to come?

"My mom sent me to you and warned me that if I stopped coming, she would cancel the generous allowance she used to give me every month."

Amazing. I did not realize he was forced to come to me. I have no idea how I would have reacted had I known the truth. However, Danny did manage to make an amazing identity change.

Nina told me she was not ready for what she experienced during the first session. She thought she was coming to a standard 45-minute appointment and found herself sitting for two hours. Throughout the meeting she wanted to go to the toilet but was too embarrassed to ask. She does not remember anything of that first meeting, except her urgent need to pee.

Brenda came to see me after her husband left her and moved in with his secretary. She told me she had three children and numerous difficulties and problems. She wanted comfort, encouragement and someone to share her sorrow with. She was shocked to find out that I asked her to make an effort. She kept coming to see me and doing her homework, but only because I told her that if she did not change she might lose her children as well. They might prefer the company of their father and his new spouse, because the atmosphere at their place was so much better. Even though our first meeting was a very long one, this possibility cut her to the quick.

Some clients do not come back after this first meeting. In the past I was bothered by that, thinking I made these people run away, and I would ask myself what else I could have done to make them cooperate. Later I found out that many of these individuals managed to make an identity change after a single meeting. The meeting gave them just the impetus they needed. This is amazing, especially as they were taught to believe that psychological therapy must be a long haul.

Despite the complexity of the first session, some clients leave my office encouraged and uplifted. They feel relieved of the burden that has oppressed them for a long time. Many of them describe their feelings in optical terms: what was foggy and blurred has become clear and distinct. The summary I provide during the meeting simplifies what had seemed so complex up until then. All of a sudden, change seems possible.

Chapter 15

The Second Meeting

Where have you been, and what have you done?

"What did you bring me?"
This is the very first question I ask my client at the second meeting. Then I take the lists he has prepared and study them thoroughly. If the client has done the homework properly, it means that items that are missing from the lists are not part of his repertoire of abilities. For example, if the word 'swimming' is not mentioned there, I assume I am dealing with a person who does not know to swim. But if at a later stage we reach the conclusion he should learn swimming, his future homework will be to acquire this ability. However, my experience has been that most clients do not include everything they were supposed to include in this initial list, although they include many unnecessary details. The list usually includes a mix of abilities, characteristics and judgments.

A person who writes that he is friendly, stubborn, sensitive, kind, conscientious, dominant and shy is not providing precise information about his abilities. These terms are meaningless generalizations whether applied to this client or to others. What is the meaning of 'sensitive'? Sensitive to what? Obviously there are areas in which the client is sensitive and areas in which he isn't. That is why detailed references stating the things people do or have done testify to their abilities much more than a list of characteristics. **Accuracy is an excellent remedy for unclear references to ourselves and to others**. When we translate generalizations into specific actions and replace judgmental evaluations with facts, a momentum of productive action will be created right from the start.

While studying the list of abilities I ask the client to clarify some items. If, for instance, he used to play the piano, I ask him how long he learned piano, and when he stopped playing. Although it was a passing episode in most cases, sometimes it turns out that the client played for many years and his ability was quite impressive. Usually I learn that the client's parents forced him to play, and when he was old enough, he quit. It is not difficult to understand that, but if his children have never listened to their father playing, it seems a tremendous waste. Let us think for a moment: What are the things we used to do in the past and no longer do? Obviously we should not consider all these things significant. Perhaps we have replaced them with better abilities. However, often people who stop an activity which is an excellent pastime fill the void created with various problems.

At this session I continue to react actively to things that arouse my interest and try to give my client some useful ideas without really knowing what will eventually influence him. I might propose, even before our survey is complete, that he brings a piano home and starts playing. By doing so, he will bring an excellent source of entertainment into the house, give his children a chance to listen to music and perhaps inspire them to learn piano too.

The first list provides us with many possibilities to start the process of evaluation and change. It is based on abilities and therefore replaces the crude, hasty diagnosis we all tend to make regarding ourselves and others. After the client replaces such diagnosis with accurate facts about his status and that of others, he will eventually reach a stage of friendly deliberation when he has to choose where to invest his energies. By writing a detailed list of abilities which are supported by real actions, the client discovers he has a rich repertoire of abilities. After he completes a proper list of abilities, he can then arrive at the answer to the question he must ask himself repeatedly on his way to change. Contrary to popular opinion, the question is not "Why am I like this?" but "Where do I stand?" When the client knows for sure where he stands, he will know, almost immediately, how to proceed. It is like reading a roadmap. Even if our map is up-to-date and clear, we won't be able to use it unless we know our exact location.

Even though my whole approach is focused on the present and the near future, it is also important to consider past abilities. We might need to use one of these dormant abilities, such as piano playing, which I have already mentioned. Every learning expert knows it is easier to reconstruct a past ability than to create a totally new one. Accordingly, before we jump into something, it is advisable for us to search our reservoir of abilities. If we find an ability we can use in order to promote change, we can channel our energies to create a new, more crucial ability.

One of the important skills I want the client to tell me about is the capacity to make friends. **The ability to make friends is one of the most important skills a person has**. On the other hand, information regarding physical appearance is irrelevant.

When we evaluate each of our abilities, we can then relate far more accurately not only to ourselves but also to others. Clients are also asked to prepare a list of abilities for some other person. Usually there is a gap between lists clients writes about themselves and lists they write about the other person — a spouse, for example. Some clients feel a little embarrassed at the second session. All of a sudden they realize they don't know much about the person who is sharing their life, and the items on the list of shared pastimes are rather limited. After I go through the list, I ask the client: "What can we learn from it?" As always, most people look for faults and indicate the things that are missing. I teach them to read more closely: "Get used to noticing the things that exist, first of all, and not the things that aren't there. The list shows you are an able person."

I do not say it just to encourage them. I simply indicate a fact that is written on the paper. The lists reveal impressive achievements that should not be taken for granted, such as studying at the Technion in Haifa, bungee-jumping, typing really fast. Moreover, the list usually provides an explanation for the problem that is disturbing the client. Anxiety, for instance, might be related to the fact that a client who was an employee all his life now has the chance to become self-employed. A couple might have reached a temporary dead-end, because before the wedding they were both absorbed in their careers and only recently, in their forties, did they get married and become parents.

It is common for clients to brandish a particular inability, difficulty or fear of a certain subject as if it were a crucial factor. I tackle this by choosing one item from the long "I can't" or "I don't like" list and suggesting it as the homework for our next meeting.

In addition, I find one significant ability on the list that I encourage the client to apply in a different context. This is a friendly act, because using an existing ability does not involve strenuous learning and is often really beneficial. Let us think for a moment: What did we use to do in the past and no longer do? Perhaps we used to play chess with our dad on Saturday mornings? If so, could we possibly play chess with our daughter now? Perhaps we earned our pocket money from painting houses as high school students. If so, maybe we could fix up our house without spending too much money.

Towards the next meeting

It's time for homework again to prepare for our third meeting. After we have gone through the list and discussed its implications, I examine the contents of the client's days: What does his day look like? What activities does it contain? What does he do during the day?

"What did you do yesterday?"
"What did you do the day before yesterday?"
"What did you do on the weekend?"

I ask the client to bring in a list of his or her daily activities. The client should write, at the end of each day, or the beginning of the next day, the activities of each day. The client should also indicate the people with whom he is sharing his time. If he just writes "Watching TV," for example, without mentioning another person, it means he did that by himself.

Sometimes, after change has already taken place, I regret not having photocopied the first list of activities, as in "before and after" ads. The first list the client brings is totally different from the lists he writes after commencing the process of change. At first he still does not know that his days will include more people and more occupations, which still leaves him some leisure time to enjoy. This usually happens when abilities improve and develop.

After assigning the homework, we move to the next topic: creating practical working tools for the production of change. I ask clients to do two kinds of homework. First of all, they should describe the days' activities in a factual way without including unnecessary information. Secondly, they should prepare a list of friendly suggestions, listing actions that are likely to improve their level of satisfaction. This list should include a wide variety of ideas, suggestions, imaginative scenarios, daring undertakings and anything else that comes to mind. I ask for 40 ideas to make sure the client has made an effort. I need him to produce an act of friendly thinking.

Sometimes I ask for more specific suggestions. If, for instance, the client complains he does not have money, I ask him to come up with various friendly suggestions to earn more money. Parents of young children who believe they do not go out much because of their children are asked to come up with 20 ideas – solutions which will enable them to go out together – a detailed list of relatives, neighbors, friends and babysitters, indicating the abilities of each to care for the children. For example, the babysitter can watch them for three hours, while grandmother can watch them for a week.

Sometimes I dispatch clients to acquire information. If, for instance, I'm dealing with a couple in crisis who are contemplating certain moves, I ask them to acquire some legal knowledge, referring them to a lawyer friend. If we are dealing with a health-related decision, I might ask for some medical tests. A person who is wavering about a business related change is asked to perform some financial consultations.

Chapter 16

The Next Meetings

So, where were we?

I examine the client's homework and check how he has spent his days. Usually, at this stage, the client already sees the homework as a friendly tool. It prevents repression, makes his days more productive and enables better use of his time.

First, I ask the client whether it was a special, or a routine week. The answer tells me whether I can use the contents for learning. Then I ask the client what can be learnt from these passing days. Here, we also refer to the items that are **missing**. For instance, if the client is a single woman who says she wants a boyfriend, I look at her homework to see whether she has dated any men. Sometimes there are no dates. All I can see is work, studying, meeting a friend, visiting parents, lots of sleep and watching TV. She spent the rest of the time alone. I ask her whether it was a typical week and she says: "Yes, it definitely was."

Obviously, there is a huge gap between what she believes she wants and what she does in practice. I ask her to add meetings and experiences with a man or several men. If she truly wants to change her identity from that of a single and find a partner, she must add many activities to her routine to help her achieve her goal. I ask her to start meeting men on a daily basis. She shouldn't delude herself that she is interested in change until she does her homework properly. Theory must become grounded in reality, and instead of constantly talking about change, she needs to make it happen. The homework should be done within a couple of days of the meeting, but not necessarily on the next day. I am a reasonable guy and do not expect her to meet seven men by our next appointment. However, I do expect her to make the first move.

My client and I build a weekly schedule, just like in any school. This time the schedule includes the friendly suggestions that we chose. After that we spend time following up their implementation and derive profit from the lessons that can be learned. I react to every inaccurate word my client says to make him aware of his previous thinking habits. For example, the unsatisfied husband says "I can't leave."
I react immediately: "Can't? Of course you can! You can go straight to the airport and travel to the other end of the world. I am not sure you should do it, but you certainly can do it."

Or, for instance, when I ask a single man about his whereabouts the previous night, he says: "I went to the movies."
"What else could you have done last night?"
"Watch TV."
"And what else?"
"Nothing. I was not in the mood to read."
"Nothing? You are absolutely sure those were the only options? A movie or watching TV?"

A single woman tells me: "I have no one to go to the movies with." I close my eyes and say: "You are not trying to see the environment. Perhaps it's difficult to find a partner and build an intimate relationship with him, but it is quite easy to find someone to go to the movies with. It is also easy to find someone who will do you a favor and sleep with you. If you post a sign on your back that says, 'Looking to hook up,' within minutes you will find a dozen volunteers."

I speak in a casual tone, but my goal is serious. I want the client to recognize her abilities and practice her outlook. She will then have the freedom of choice that will enable her to shape her identity even before the infrastructure of sharpened thinking tools is completed.

Getting to work – Beginning change

So far I have gathered information about the client, and more importantly, taught him to gather information about himself. By now the client also knows how to gather information, rather than judgments, about other people in his life – his wife, his children, his associates.

It's time for change. Since it is only the beginning, we start with a small change in an insignificant area. The experiment will be completed within a short period of time, a day or a weekend. Tom, for example, is a teenager who hates school, especially history lessons. He was asked to find interesting articles on the Internet dealing with historical topics. My goal was to cure him of his aversion to the subject. Karen, who was afraid to ride a bicycle, was taught the basics of riding in a short course. At the end of the course, given by a friend of hers, she started to enjoy the new skill she acquired and felt more confident in her ability to make changes.

That's it – the tools have been sharpened, and we have already managed to make a small change. It is time for bigger changes. The client and I get ready for all possible scenarios, but unpredictable things happen from time to time. I am available to my clients day and night, and they do not hesitate to call. I recall, for example, Maria's desperate phone call. She was trying to develop her relationship with her partner and move in with him. She prepared a draft in advance where she wrote the things she wanted to tell him, and we edited this text together several times. In our telephone conversation Maria told me she had an opportunity to talk to him, and that he had reacted with total rejection.

"Everything is lost," she said.

"Lost? Maybe not," I reassured her and told her it was a predictable, instinctive reaction. It did not necessarily reflect the actions her boyfriend might take a few days after her words had sunk in. Meanwhile, she was to move to plan B, put an ad in the paper that she was looking for a roommate and start interviewing interested male candidates.

Maria calmed down and did as I said. A week later her boyfriend realized that she was not going to wait for him forever, and that she might form a relationship with the roommate she selected. He started making moves to improve their relationship.

The week of change is very crucial. These are the days during which change is produced. Afterwards all we need to do is to keep it on the right track. A few weeks later the change will become part of our identity.

Change in the eyes of the client

It is very difficult to catch the moment when the change occurs. When does a person know a change has taken place? In most cases people first start to function differently, and then they gradually realize that they have changed. However, sometimes they become aware of the change immediately.

Ross came to see me because he had experienced great difficulties with his wife for a whole year. They were married for two years and had a baby, but he felt as if his whole world had collapsed and blamed her. The minute he came home his wife started complaining and demanding things, attacking him like a vampire. She was wicked, evil. He had to defend himself constantly, feeling weaker and weaker, losing his lust for life. He felt like a squeezed lemon. This nightmare repeated itself every evening. She seemed ugly, repulsive and scary. He started fantasizing about a magical solution – he could just kill her. A wonderful solution indeed. If she was dead, everything would be great. The only problem is that he might be locked up in a prison cell for the rest of his life, but he could prevent it by planning the perfect crime. This decision made him feel better, that there was light at the end of the tunnel. At this point he came to see me.

At the second meeting I changed everything for him in just one sentence: "What do you want from the poor woman? You make her look like a monster. You have plenty of abilities, but now you're acting in an infantile manner. Do something to change the situation."

All the hatred he felt was gone in a second. He saw her as she really was. On that day he came home with a new perspective, a fresh outlook and reacted to his wife almost affectionately. Previously he had only been aware of how his wife made him feel, and all of a sudden he managed to see **her** – all day at home with the baby, without any help and feeling exhausted. Then, when she turned to her husband, he was not really there. The way to change had been paved.

Sharon described something else. One day we were reviewing the previous week's activity report, which was similar to the ones before and contained bad, depressing days.

I said, "Do something nice for yourself. Fill your days with activities you enjoy. Spend some time with people you like. Make sure to defy your limits and focus on things you like and enjoy."

"Why didn't you tell me all this before?" she asked.

In fact, I had told her that, time and again. I said, "I have been telling you that for ages."

I do not know why she suddenly realized she was the one who was responsible for her days and that she could shape them as she liked. She is like the person who came into my office and said "That new picture you bought is really nice," when in fact it had hung there for a few years. The picture had been there all along, but he only noticed it on that day.

Bradley felt good at work and bad at home with his wife and children. I told him two things to promote the process of change. The first thing was the way I described my relationship with my wife and children. I told him it was a source of pleasure and that, for me, home was the most pleasant place. It was not the words I used that made him want to be in a similar situation, but rather my warm intonation when describing the situation at my house. The second thing that triggered change was my declaration that in Friendship School, abilities are binding. In certain areas he had to do all he could, not only what he felt like.

That evening, when he came home, his wife immediately demanded that he prepare a salad. He wanted to rest a little, but had to admit that the salad his wife was asking him to prepare was, surprisingly enough, something he was capable of doing. Then he wanted to watch TV, but his son called him over. Usually, when his children called upon him, the tone of his reaction would make them leave him alone for the rest of the evening. This time he stood up – ability is binding, I had said – and asked his son what he wanted.

At the end of the day he lay in bed, exhausted, when all of a sudden his wife started fondling him, probably because he had behaved differently that evening. He knew that by saying just a few words, he could make her turn away, insulted, but he came to his senses, and although he did not really want to, he responded. The long day had not ended yet. It was an exhausting day.

The next day was not much different, and he felt that his efforts were almost too much for him. Still, he forced himself to go on. After a few such evenings he told himself: "If I can't do as I like, maybe I'll try to enjoy what I am doing." It was as if he had flipped a switch in his brain. The change was remarkable. The next evenings were similar to the previous ones, but now he did not feel exhausted and empty at the end of the day. On the contrary, he felt animated and amused and had an appetite for more. Bradley describes it as a significant turning point in his life. The evenings he spends with his family have become the highlight of his days.

Allen's parents were concerned. Their son was a client of mine, and they thought that the reason he came to me was his low self-esteem and his lack of success with girls. During his military service, Allen worked with computers, and after his discharge he started working at a high-tech company. The parents were concerned about the fact that their son did not want to study at university and expected me to encourage him to do so. The first meeting was confrontational, since I gave my opinion that their son was doing the right thing and his studies could wait.

At first his mother was assertive and determined, but eventually both parents changed their attitude and became friendly. Later, the mother told me she changed her attitude after hearing that I had visited their son at his workplace. Before approaching him, I watched him and saw him standing in front of many people, mostly older than himself, giving a presentation about a topic I was unfamiliar with. Once he finished, the listeners started asking questions and requesting further explanations. It turned out that their son was a whiz in this field. I mentioned the high salary he earned, despite his young age, and said that perhaps he did not need to study since he knew so much. I was convinced that just as he had learned everything he needed to learn so far, he would continue to develop in the future, and if he believed academic studies would help, he would apply to university.

However it was not my rational arguments that convinced the mother. What influenced her was that before expressing my opinion I performed a learning activity – I visited him at his workplace. She blushed from embarrassment, since it would never have occurred to her to find out exactly where he worked, and what he actually did. All she knew was that he was not a university student and that it wasn't right.

***

Do the descriptions written above help us understand something? Maybe, and maybe not. This is an arbitrary collection of answers my clients gave me when I asked them what made them change. No one really knows the mysteries of the human brain, and change requires constant searching and a creative approach.

Chapter 17

The Partner Gets Involved

What does your partner say about this?

When I was still practicing clinical psychology and was not bothered by reality, I would accompany patients into the therapeutic bubble where we analyzed their feelings, emotions, memories and dreams. Today, my focus is on reality. Though I am aware that the client is very important, I also take into account the other people that live with him – spouse, children, perhaps parents. The client's welfare depends on their welfare, and any change that is triggered will also change something for them. That is why I feel I should take them into consideration. Only when the spouse or other family members refuse to cooperate do I interact exclusively with the client.

Sometimes the problem is not a lack of cooperation from the spouse, but the fact that the spouse is unaware of our meetings. In general, I do not agree to a situation where a woman meets with me without telling her husband, since I believe it compromises her identity. If she is afraid to tell her husband this simple fact, how can she possibly make more significant changes? She does not need to ask for his permission before meeting a psychologist she trusts (or a gynecologist, or other professional) but only to inform him of her intentions. Psychological therapy is not like an expensive new car, which should be bought only after the couple makes a mutual decision. However, I realize that at the beginning, were the wife to inform the husband, he would either give me credit for all the changes, or hold them against me, while continuing to see his wife in the same light. That is why I sometimes agree to hold two or three more sessions without the husband's knowledge, just until the first series of changes is underway. By then the status quo has shifted, which might induce him to cooperate.

Anyway, when I recognize the first signs that my client intends to make a change, I ask to meet the spouse so as to disturb the family balance as little as possible. "Ask your husband if he can meet me once, free of charge," I request, stressing that I need only one meeting. I say this in order not to give the husband the impression of being dragged into something he is not interested in. I will convince him to cooperate only if he too is likely to benefit. I also emphasize that no payment is necessary so that he won't feel that I am inviting him for the wrong reasons.

In the previous chapter I wrote about male clients, but here my emphasis is deliberately on female clients. Women tend to accept changes in their husbands more easily. Changes in the wife, even positive ones, might be perceived as burdens by her spouse. It is one thing for the wife to start working outside the house, but God forbid if she starts making more money than the husband. In many cases the husband will even try to interfere in the process.

If the husband agrees to meet me, I usually explain that his wife came to see me because she wanted to make a change, which I think she is capable of doing. I add that I do not know exactly where the change will lead. Then I ask him two questions. First I ask for his version, or how he sees the scenery. So far I have heard the woman's version, but now I'm interested to hear his. Then I ask: if you could place an order for certain character traits and physical appearance where your wife is concerned, what would you request? If he is a nice man and loves his wife, I have nothing to add. I know for sure that we can count on his cooperation. The woman is lucky to have her spouse as a friend. However, this type of friendship is not that common. In most cases the husband starts complaining about the wife, says he would like her to change, that he does not need to change, nor does he see the need to invest in their relationship.

At this point I sometimes pose a provocative question: "Would it bother you if you knew your wife had slept with another man?"

If the husband's answer reflects a lack of interest in his wife or even a wish to get rid of her, I pose another question: "Does the thought that your children will sit on another man's lap bother you?"

These two questions are my attempt to increase the man's scope of vision beyond the tip of his nose. Time and again I come across short-sighted people who make fatal moves, and who are shocked when they realize the possible outcomes of their actions. My questions do not mean I know in advance what will happen in their relationship. However, the scenario I show him is very likely. I pose a few additional provocative questions. Such questions are sometimes needed to shake up a person and make him work harder. Let us take, for example, a man who intends to leave his home and maybe move in with a girlfriend. He has a clear picture of the life awaiting him, without considering any effects of this move on his wife, his older daughter or his son. Before he makes his move, I try, making myself brutally clear, to apprise him of other possible scenarios so he will consider the eventual cost of his actions. Perhaps his daughter will not forgive him, and the friendship between father and daughter will become hostility? Perhaps his son will do something horrible to himself? I don't intend to deter him from making the move. Some moves are worthwhile no matter what. I can even help him realize his plan while minimizing the damage as much as possible. True, he is not my client, but I want him to visualize the future clearly and see beyond his short-sightedness.

Many people take these questions seriously, saying clearly they do not want to lose what they have. I suggest they stay in touch with me. Perhaps they will join their spouse for two or three sessions to make sure any personal changes suit both of them. Other men just laugh in my face. They know their wives well and know how little they are capable of. If so, I make no suggestions.

Anyhow, I thank them for coming and say goodbye.

Martha – A case study

Forty-year-old Martha came to see me. She looked terribly exhausted. She was a homemaker, married to a widower. He had brought his two grownup children into the marriage and, in addition, they had three children together. It was a very difficult time for her as her husband was having an affair. Although he had not moved out, he ignored his wife altogether. His children did not respect her and were a burden to her, while their father always backed them up. She had undergone unsuccessful psychological therapy and was now about to tell me about her miserable life in detail.

At the very first session I told her I would not listen to her complaints about her husband and his children because she was the one who allowed them to act that way. "If you act like a housemaid, why should they treat you differently? You are totally predictable, and it's no wonder they take you for granted. The only significant question we will discuss during our sessions is whether you can change. If it turns out you can, it will be interesting to see what changes will take place in your family."

Martha listened to me, nodded, and went home determined to make a change.

During our talk I learned that she had had an important positon in the army, and that she had learned guitar for a few years before giving up music. She used to work outside the house but quit after giving birth. Her previous psychological therapy had lasted for two years and focused on her husband's infidelity. From reports of how she spent her days, I learned that she devoted most of her time to providing various services – preparing meals for everybody, serving the meals and cleaning the table. She spent the evenings by herself. Her husband watched TV with his children or went out on his own, while she was bitter and full of complaints. When she looked at her reports, she started laughing at herself: "How did I become such a drudge?"

After our next session, when I sensed that Martha was ready for change, I invited her husband separately. When he arrived, I asked him for his version and let him speak for a few minutes. She was unattractive, complained and bugged everyone. He was forced to defend his children because she did not love them. They were sensitive and had already been through traumas, and he had already taken them to psychologists.

I told him that Martha was going to change soon. I said I could not predict the direction of the changes: perhaps she would leave him, or become acquainted with another man and take their children along with her. He laughed out loud and reassured me, "You've nothing to worry about. I've known her for many years. She came to cry on your shoulder, but she isn't really capable of doing anything. She is totally dependent on me. I wish she would start moving."

This time I informed Martha of the things he had said, though I don't always do that. My report confirmed her suspicion that she was perceived as a predictable person, but made her even more determined to continue. However, she brought a rather limited list of suggestions for change. We picked out one of them – the guitar. Martha brought a guitar home, and her children, who heard her play for the first time, sang along with her. Soon they asked for guitar lessons.

The list also contained a few suggestions related to jobs, so that she could earn some money and would not be totally dependent on her husband when she wanted to buy something. She found a part-time job in a shop in town. She started going out at night, and her freedom of movement slowly increased. First she went to visit friends, then she started enjoying herself even more. When the shop owner started flirting with her, Martha responded. They had a small pleasant fling.

For many years Martha believed that once she was able to go out and enjoy life, she would divorce her husband, demand high alimony for the three children and live happily without him. It did not turn out that way. The shocked husband started wooing his wife vigorously – trips abroad, gifts and similar inducements – a kind of second honeymoon. Martha concluded that this alternative was much friendlier than her other option of single parenthood and partial relationships, so she started seriously investing in her marriage.

Together or apart?

I conduct meetings with both spouses only when the spouses are friends who cooperate in the process of change. I won't be caught in the midst of a conflict. In such a situation, they are not available for negotiation. They irritate one another, and I cannot possibly do any good. On the other hand, when the spouses are friends, they complete one another and add to one another. They, as a couple, have a reservoir of abilities which enables them to produce as many changes as they like. Their mutual view is much more comprehensive than their separate views. When a couple invests all their efforts in producing change, success will undoubtedly follow.

Harry and Ruth, parents of a little girl, used to fight a lot. Their stormy quarrels led to frequent separations, but they always got back together till the next fight. Despite their conflicts, I felt that they could work together and produce change. Their invariable reunions and the fact that they chose to come to me together gave the impression that the force holding them together was stronger than the force tearing them apart. Do you recall the language of facts?

Their personal texts were extremely predictable, repeated by each until they knew them verbatim: "He is twice-divorced, so obviously he has a problem," "Her parents always used to." I suggested they put their egocentrism aside and start considering others, such as their daughter and each other. I also said that in times of conflict each one must find a way to prevent the approaching fight. Even if only one of them acted this way, the goal would be achieved. They offered some examples which we used to examine retrospectively and discuss what could have been done to prevent a fight.

We also decided they would change their previous habits and draw up new rules. From now on, the minute they felt rising hostility that prevented them from enjoying their time together, they would go their separate ways for a couple of hours. This was another way to prevent quarrels. When they were tired of each other, the short separation would enable them to rest a little and then go back without needing to fight. As a challenge, I suggested that if they did wind up fighting and separating for a longer period of time, they should not sit idly by, waiting for the next reconciliation, but go out and have fun with other partners. This way they would both feel the threat if they allowed themselves to fight as they used to.

In addition, I offered them two tips: First, I advised them to do a lot of physical activity, such as walking together and separately, and secondly, I suggested that in the next couple of weeks they should plan their meetings and not just be spontaneous. I pointed out that recently, when they tried to spend time together spontaneously, they tended to fight over nonsense. Sometimes he wanted to come home, find a dish that was prepared especially for him, put his feet on the table and watch TV, while she expected to go out to eat. She got mad because they didn't go out, and he got mad because he was hungry. The net result was a fierce fight.

During the next couple of days they practiced their homework. Sometimes one of them called me for some encouragement. I accompanied the process during four or five sessions and that was it. They embarked on a second honeymoon. I suggested that they should keep their relationship on this track and add even more special amusements occasionally. I truly hope they took my advice.

Winding up our meetings

Most people need two or three intensive meetings to prepare and equip themselves for change, and a few practical hands-on meetings during which I accompany them through the actual process of change. When clients get on the right track, they proceed by themselves and no longer need me. Others occasionally come in for a meeting where they summarize what they have managed so far, and we think over the next steps.

There are a few clients who prefer to meet me on a regular basis. They are obviously affluent enough to do so and want me to be part of their support network. I agree to regular meetings only if the clients are not burdensome. I refer here to clients who are constantly developing, avoid dwelling on the same subject and do not use our sessions to reinforce unfriendly habits. When these routine meetings disrupt the process of growth, or I see no further readiness to change, I feel obliged to put a stop to these sessions too.

Chapter 18

Some Parting Words

In this book I have introduced some remarkable and unique tools. However, I would like to emphasize again that it is not enough just to understand these tools. They require extensive and repeated practice. Some people who are trapped by the stifling culture of canonical psychology will find it hard to keep going for a long period of time. Others, who can see all the options, discover that their mission is possible and even easy to accomplish. On the personal level, it is most important not to dwell on so-called problems, but concentrate on abilities and issues that can be promoted and are worth promoting. If we choose to do this, the problems will automatically resolve themselves.

It is not only ourselves that we are able to change, but also our relationships with others. In fact, we change our environment from the moment we are born, whether or not we intend to do so. However, it is during adolescence that we are able to produce change intentionally and logically for the first time. Though we discussed adolescence only from the parental viewpoint, in practice, adolescents are able to change their 'stuck' parents and even their younger siblings. Actually, some adolescents do so without any prompting. They introduce new data and by doing so start a chain of changes. At the adult stage, those who are interested in changing their relationship with a partner can develop the necessary abilities and use them within the relationship. Similarly, parents can produce changes in their young children or adolescents. The most important thing is not to drag children and teenagers to unproductive psychological therapies or diagnoses.

We can also change other areas of our lives. We can learn to make the most of our jobs, to improve our health, to adjust to changes that were forced upon us, such as retirement or children leaving home. On the whole, we can change throughout our lives if we develop a wide perspective or outlook. As members of the learning culture, we will never become smug. We will always realize how minimal our ability is compared to the abundance of stimuli that beckon us and be aware that our current knowledge is insufficient. Our endless journey will expose us to information that will constantly change the fixed patterns in our brain.

In this book I have focused on the changes we go through as individuals, but change is significant and relevant too where broader systems are concerned. In the workplace, employees can make extensive changes if they get together and wield their power. The educational system has enough resources to work wonders and easily correct parents' naïve mistakes, if it were only more adept and less conservative. A professional system that focuses on nurturing abilities, instead of labeling and categorizing students, could create a variety of growth opportunities.

Canonical psychology must change. Admittedly, analytic thinking sometimes has its uses. Locating the source of the problem in a car's engine, for example, immediately leads to an effective solution.

Obviously, approaches and techniques do not need to change in garages where cars are being repaired. However, psychology must get rid of its traditional thinking habits. Treating felons and mental patients could be much more effective if the system were not based on outmoded psychological methods. Nowadays individuals are still categorized by titles such as 'drug addicts,' 'violent offenders' or 'schizophrenics' and treated accordingly. All the rehabilitation and drug-prevention programs that are implemented for criminals are doomed to failure. They only force people to deal with more sophisticated challenges. Therapeutic and rehabilitation programs for mental patients are also doomed to failure. I can say with authority that this group needs to develop important abilities, as I have made inroads in this particular area. The state can maintain its authority and keep criminals and mental patients in closed institutions, but it must treat them differently. Instead of accelerating the decline of these institutions, in which criminals become more professional and mental patients deteriorate, it should transform them into places where various activities that promote personal abilities take place, and where identity changes can be made. The final system is the government, as mentioned earlier. It is rather depressing to think what awesome changes it could have produced were it not so short-sighted. This is because it is focused on achieving the personal goals of politicians who do not consider the public welfare.

I would like to believe that someday my method will be taught even in kindergarten. Learning the basics of friendly thinking during infancy is enjoyable and helps the ability to think clearly develop. When children become older, their thinking already follows fixed patterns and is hard to change.

Sadly, the existence of our whole world today depends on leaders with rigid thinking and beliefs who have the power to destroy it. Our existence should not be taken for granted. In order to minimize the many dangers we face, we must get used to the learning culture from a young age. I am not preaching about values but about developing our ability to survive. This might sound unrealistic, but if the momentum for change gets underway, we will certainly succeed.

As it stands, unfortunately, most of us were not educated about the learning culture in our early years. That is why we should remind ourselves repeatedly that the ability to change is a right to which we are all entitled. In order to exercise this right, we must be capable of choosing between as many alternatives as possible. Nowadays, freedom of choice is still not considered a must. Most people struggle for it because they have not acquired it naturally through standard educational processes. **An act of learning is the only way we can change feelings and emotions fixed in place by previous habits. We must go out and fight for our right to change. We should take advantage of all available methods, including sophisticated and complex ones, on our way to achieving this goal!**

Glossary

My Glossary ....
Ability ....
Blocking ....
Brain ....
Brain Meetings ....
Bypass ....
Causality ....
Compensation ....
Concentration ....
Constraint ....
Crude Rejection ....
Culture Pocket ....
Days' content ....
Dealing with "problems" Delinquency ....
Depression ....
Developing / Developmental Bug ....
Enforcement Tools ....
Entertaining Quality ....
Friendly Thinking ....
Friendship ....
Homework ....
Identity ....
Immediate Relief ....

Junction of Opportunities
Language of Communication
Leakage
Learning Culture
Learning Decliner
Learning Workshops
"Low Self Image
Management
Maximal Reduction
Mental Budget
Opportunity
Production
Public Opinion
Quarrels
Relevant Stimulus
Repression
Satisfaction
Scenery
Sensational Diagnosis
State of Aggregation
Symptom
Technology
Trampled Culture (Culture of Diagnosis & Judgment
Work Meetings

My Glossary

During the years in which I worked as a psychologist I have sensed an increasing dissatisfaction with the language of psychology and philosophy. Awkward and general concepts do not suit the ones who wish to study and get to know people and seek innumerable ways to produce friendly changes. Thus, I have found myself producing terms that appropriately express my professional attitude and the modus operandi of the "Friendship School" I have founded. The need for producing these terms arises from my wish to avoid using treatment, medical and deterministic concepts. I cannot possibly conceal my pretence of creating a thinking language that seems to me as an appropriate language for dealing with people and of taking advantage of their living space within a constrained, rigid world of data. Some of the terms were coined by me, and some were borrowed. I do not make do with a mere literal interpretation of the various concepts. In order to facilitate the understanding of 'friendly thinking' and its implementation in practice, I chose to write in detail about many of the concepts. The concepts touch upon each other, and are sometimes overlapping and interwoven, since developing friendly thinking tools is not an organized, structured process. Therefore, although they are written one after the other, one should see them as though they were written next to each other. It is not easy to change fixed thinking patterns. Be patient with yourself until you acquire tools which will be further sharpened through experiences and you will develop a clear perception, **which will become extremely useful**. I recommend using this glossary as food for a journey and also as home port to which you can return from time to time in order to digest what you have met throughout our mutual voyages.

Ability

Everything we do today, everything we did in the past and everything we will be able to do in the future.

In fact, ability is a molecule of <u>identity</u>: It is a kind of secured, accurate anchorage in a sea of imaginary versions and assumptions – the expectations, crude diagnosis, opinions and judgments that a person operates upon himself and others. All of these things are abstract and difficult to measure and only the things we do in practice reflect truthfully the things we are able to do.

This is a reliable but not necessarily exhaustive forecast. Many people miss the opportunity to demonstrate their ability thoroughly.

Selecting the reservoir of abilities of a person is choosing accurate, reliable data on condition that the person does not repress his abilities. You cannot add another meter to yourself. This is indeed an inability. All other things are things you cannot do at the moment or things you are not in the mood to do at the moment. A person who does not make a distinction between a sense of inability and real inability is doomed to pay a high price. **Repression of ability** causes the greatest damage. Such a person is like a blind person who is unable to enjoy the colors of the world or a deaf person who cannot hear sounds. The damage in this case is to the brain. The person **feels** he is unable and acts as if he really is. However, when we manage to get rid of the curtain of repressing abilities, the abilities are exposed immediately one by one. A picture of a person who finally discovers his abilities is a very moving one.

On the other hand, people who are part of the scholastic culture do not repress their abilities. On the contrary, they continue to develop. They add more and more to the system of abilities – and shape their identity accordingly. They can promote certain ability on account of another and make changes in their identity. A person who learns how to drive changes his identity from a pedestrian to a driver. A single man who learnt to live with a woman becomes a spouse. A person who separated from a woman and lives by himself becomes a bachelor again.

The identity contains our abilities in different states of aggregations. **Investing in learning processes changes and shapes our identity.** Our ability flows in the channels of expression. As water flows in the rivers and the streams, the capable person drains his abilities into a certain channel towards a person who needs them. This is a top to bottom movement. From the "more" to the "less." There is someone who recognizes he has something to add to another person or to a certain subject. When we are incapable in a certain area, we constitute a possibility for a capable person who can contribute to us. (The most fascinating production is a friendly production in which two people identify what they can add to each other and how they can enjoy each other; and beyond it, a community of friends).

In a **trampled culture** the channel of ability is fixated in an unchanging pattern in which everything flows in the same courses all the time. On the other hand, in a scholastic culture, everything moves in fascinating growth processes which create a changing variety of combinations of relationships of people; abilities flow from one vessel to the other and everybody **learns and teaches at the same time.** I refer to **feelings and emotions** as an expression of ability. Every person feels and senses the things he is used to feel and sense. An individual who does only the things he likes to do, remains the same – he only recycles himself and becomes totally predictable. A person who knows how to learn, knows how to add new abilities to himself. First he acquires the basis of ability and if he is persistent in the learning process, he will turn into a proficient expert.

The shaping of identity might take place even without a sense of desire and eagerness. A person might reach an arbitrary decision since he understands the advantages of change and succeed in making the change.

Changing our feeling is at the top of our learning ability. This is the fruit of investment of people who are persistent in their learning. Of course there is no need to change everything and it is also impossible. If, for instance, someone has been shaving the same way for ages, there is no need for him to change it. On the other hand, if he likes a certain kind of music, and despises more up-to-date music, he should, perhaps, make an effort and learn how to prick up his ears so that he will be able to enjoy music with his children in the present or in the future.

In scholastic culture ability is compelling! This is the true basis for friendly homework. Doing what you can. No more, but no less. This is the reliable foundation for making changes in our identity, at the top of which a deep, thorough emotional change takes place. It should be mentioned that a deep emotional change is not achieved merely by doing. It is achieved mainly by paying undivided attention to the doing and concentrating on it. For example, it is not enough to listen to background music, you must really concentrate on it until you internalize it and it becomes part of you, becomes really yours. See: "Identity"

Blocking

Sealing of the brain which eliminates curiosity and ability to choose and promotes a totally predictable, predefined way of life. Being born in the right place at the right time is a matter of luck. In the past, when society was more traditional and closed the identity of most people was shaped in advanced: they were born, as blocked people, into a very narrow world and spent their entire life there. That used to be the common social reality. Since the world was sparsely populated and transportation and communication means were limited, the contact with other cultures was minimal. Most people never left their village and had the same occupation throughout their lifetime; they acted as if the world outside their world did not exist. Blockings can also be created nowadays by a person who lives amongst us but for some reason is unable to enjoy his life. He is tensed, exhausted and suffering so he decides to minimize his world awkwardly and retires to an island of rest from the burden of life. In most cases he will choose to join one of the already existing culture pockets or to create a minimized world for himself. **Such a person behaves as if he is not surrounded by a world full of stimulations.** He does not sense, he does not feel, does not want or need anything else. Where there is no desire – there is no pain. When there are not any stimulations, there are not any symptoms. He lives in a type of dungeon and does not need anything. In most cases he lives in total solitary or close to people who live like him, in the same minimized world; people who do not "threaten" to expose him to the things he is unable to contain.

Such a person usually feels well since there is no gap between his capabilities and the contents of his world. He does not have the will to experience and broaden his world. As time passes by, the huge gap that has been created between him and people of other culture serves as an efficient, protective wall. The effort required for bridging the gaps is so enormous that he prefers to remain at the same, familiar place.

Thus, a blocking is a cultural event related to the brain. There are many examples of these **culture pockets**: a homogeneous religious group that dissociates itself from the rest of society such as a mystic cult or an Indian ashram; new immigrants who live in a community of people from the same country and do not learn the new language or the new culture; ultra-orthodox Jews who devote all their time to learning the Torah in a secluded society; obedient followers of a certain political party; people who devote all their time to their work; people who suffer from chronic depression, old people in a parents home and so forth. When a blocking exists the person controls his world; in fact, he recycles himself fanatically. He is free from the dynamics of the constant friction with a cultural society full of stimulations which is ever-changing and requires constant learning.

Blocking can serve as a successful solution to people who feel good and protected in a limiting setting. But – and here is the weak point of blocking – the solution is successful as long as the person does not feel the urge to get out of the box, and as long as stimulations do not invade it. Such a person perceives all types of change as negative; changes make him suffer and lead to extremely awkward reactions. He must react with <u>crude rejection</u>. As our eyes respond to a grain of sand.

The most difficult position is the position of people who have "fell between two stools." For instance, someone who has left the convenient religious pocket but does not allow himself to enjoy the secular freedom. He is in no man's land: he does not feel well here, and does not feel well there. Or someone who decides to narrow down his world but has not created an efficient partitioning between himself and the world around him. Let's take for example a woman who decides to live on her own without roommates or male friends. All she wants is to study. But she lives in the big city and the sounds of life around her ring out. From time to time she experiences pockets of silence, when she shuts herself in her room, reading a book. But when she goes out of the apartment she is surrounded by hugging couples. She then finds out that a schoolmate of hers got married, that another friend of hers had a baby. she finds it unbearable. Surely it is easier to be a secluded nun on a top of a mountain or to live with other nuns at the monastery.

Thus, an awkward minimization of one's world also requires some efforts in order to be successful. And it gets more and more difficult as time goes by, population grows and contact with the rest of the world becomes inevitable. The media which is everywhere – from newspapers and TV to internet and cellular phones – makes it difficult to create a blocked ghetto.

Brain

The most important and missed organ of human beings.
Our attitude towards our eyes, the organs of sight, is much better than our attitude towards our brain. We do everything we can possibly do in order to see well, we notice when our sight is faulty and we use eye glasses in order to make it better. But only a few people bother to nurture their organ of thinking and identity and improve its ability as much as possible. The situation is grave since many people believe their brain functions perfectly. Not even a single section in their brain examines their way of thinking even when it leads them to faulty considerations and even when they make the same mistakes over and over again. They let their brain function like other internal organs such as the spleen or the pancreas and invest in their body but never in their brain. Some boast of numerous sensitivities and allergies and remove allergenic substances from their surroundings so that they will not get a rash, or snuffles or skin irritation God forbid! But they do not have mercy on their brain. They burden it with drugs, alcohol, and perhaps, worst of all, flood it with perfect nonsense and silly superstitions. So that every so often a thinking person sticks out as a lighthouse in a sea of fools.

Developing the brain means developing friendly thinking as a navigator. Some people believe that the brain is separated from the emotions or the soul, and that the development of the brain promotes only the brain. In fact, the real separation is between the feelings and thoughts of a person who remains in kindergarten and a person who grows and develops. The brain is also an organ of emotions so its nurturing through sharpening the tools of thinking, concentration and attention enriches the emotional life as well. Nevertheless, our orientation through our senses and emotions is very problematic. It is true that our brain knows how to understand information that contradicts our direct senses. For instance, we see that the sun revolves around earth, but most of us know today that it is not so and that earth revolves around the sun. A naked eye cannot see bacteria, but we know they exist. (It should be mentioned though that these discoveries were not accepted easily and willingly. Some scientists even lost their lives while struggling with swarms of raging people who believed blindly in the Holy Scriptures, religious scholars and illiterate crowds).

But, in general, most people are still convinced that their emotions reflect reality. In most cases it is not so. For example, mourning for many years over the loss of a dear one does not necessarily reflect deep feelings or great love. On the contrary, it is a testimony to shabby feelings. A person who is rich in feelings will mourn his loss for a while, for instance, a bereaved father mourns the death of his son for a while and then he is excited again about his other children and not so excited about the loss of that child. A woman who keeps mourning the death of her father instead of channeling her love towards her spouse and her children is in fact crudely rejecting the relevant elements in her life through mourning. Approaches that stand for mourning processing and support groups for terror victims, second and third generation of holocaust survivors and the likes seem unfriendly to me since they turn the mourning into a routine pastime. In Friendship School we make a clear distinction between events and habits, language and pastime. The event is accompanied by a traumatic experience and we offer first aid by all means. But before the person becomes an addict we try to move on. A person should be cautious about an addiction to suffering as he is cautious about an addiction to morphine.

See: "Friendly Thinking."

Brain Meetings

The two or three first meetings between the client and myself in which we pinpoint the current position of the client and discuss the things he should do in order to promote himself.

During these meetings the guide is supposed to study the clients and especially to study what they have gained so far, what brings them to the Friendship School and what they should acquire in the process. The client is supposed to learn the language of friendly thinking, to sharpen his brain and to create tools which will be useful for shaping his identity or changing his previous one.

People who are used to sessions with an attentive therapist, sometimes find it difficult to get used to a more active style. In my books I refer to such a person as "therapy damaged." It takes time until he understands that the homework is there **for his sake** and not for the therapist's sake. In the past he was encouraged to talk about his feelings to his wife or other present or past relatives. It took a long time and his money contributed a great deal to the clinical therapist's bank account. The homework might impose a burden on the client and irritate him, but it is highly efficient and promotes him. From time to time someone stands up and walks away during the very first meeting. People ask me why I burden the applicants with homework. A person who finds it difficult to do relatively simple homework, should not be misled into thinking that he is about to make much more complex, complicated changes.

In general, I try to schedule the brain meetings so that one meeting follows the previous one and there are no long time gaps between them in order to create a mass of impact in the direction of change. Later, once change is produced, the meetings can be either reduced or stopped altogether. The whole process can be quick and amazingly efficient.

Sometimes I give the applicants a handout which says:

In Friendship School you start a process of **learning, enrichment, counseling and guidance.** You will go through experiences which are a sort of "homework." This is clearly not a clinical psychological therapy. Here you cannot be a patient. You come here in order to sharpen your thinking tools and learn how to produce changes which will be beneficial in numerous areas of life.

Producing a change is not the result of constant dwelling on the problems, but of adding abilities which we will select together.

I must make an apology. A person who gets here by accident and is not familiar with <u>friendly thinking</u>, or has not read my books before, will probably experience considerable difficulty. He is expected to come across things which contradict the things he has known for ages. He might get upset and annoyed. Someone else might get hurt although my intention is not to hurt but to trigger thought.

In Friendship School, contrary to traditional psychology, we do not deal with detailed descriptions of feelings and emotions. Instead, we suggest referring to the things that the client **has done** so far or **is still doing**. The language of **facts** is much more reliable and accurate than opinions and judgments. It is worthwhile to learn how to scan the scenery we are constantly exposed to and to discover that we are capable of adding more and more abilities to our reservoir. This type of learning grants us the ability to choose.

I am convinced that adequate reference to people requires thinking tools which are different from the popular ones.

You should **be very patient with yourselves** until you are able acquire more sophisticated and creative tools.

You will find out that you do not come only "to pour out your troubles" and talk non-stop. You can do that free of charge with your neighbor. **You come in order to hear and listen as well**. Moreover, you will find out that at first the talks sound as if the subjects are changed arbitrarily. At first it makes it difficult to concentrate since most people are used to rational, organized thinking and to forming preconceptions which prevent them from seeing most of the scenery. We will try to train you to scan a broad scenery without forcing arbitrary organization.

In addition to the meetings, it is recommended to read Rafi Yaakobby's books and the friendly lexicon which can be found at the archives of the Friendship School site.

If you do not understand something – ask! If you have comments or complaints – **react!** Where? During sessions or by email. Moreover, you can use the questions section on the internet site.

Bypass

A course in which we bypass the SYMPTOM or the "problematic" element, force ourselves to do what we can and move determinedly towards a friendly goal.

This term refers to the practical aspect of producing change. A person who is interested in change is required to make a crucial decision and choose one of two approaches. The common, most popular approach is that of the therapeutic culture – namely the medical, psychological and psychiatric culture: a problem is diagnosed, and taken care of. According to this order; the problem must be fixed first and only afterwards it is possible to move on. Huge efforts are made during therapy which is dedicated to crude rejections means, namely, to dealing with "problems."

Most people truly believe that as long as they do not overcome anxiety, sorrow or suffering – it is not possible to move on. They believe that after they finish taking care of all of their problems, a day will come and everything will be good. Sometimes, a person who tries to find another channel for finding solutions is considered a coward who runs away from his problems. As far as I am concerned, this is how we become enslaved by a damaging occupation which is totally unfriendly. I truly believe that a person who is treated by a doctor, namely an officer of medicine, is bound to become sicker and sicker; a person who is treated by a psychologist who diagnoses and catalogs people and encourages them to speak about their problems is bound to become a patient who suffers from cerebral and identity damage. "I am like that!" in the sense that I cannot be changed and if such a person tries to change he will content himself with little, as a person who has been diagnosed as a retard is contented with understanding first grade arithmetic. Indeed it is possible that his suffering and pains disappear as time goes by and it is good enough for him. It is enough for him. He does not expect to feel real good or happy.

But, in most cases, people who are used to live their lives that way, keep feeling the things they are used to feel, namely, they will replace one pain with another or one problem with other problems.

Most therapeutic approaches are terribly narrow-minded since the therapists ignore two important facts. First, their patient is much more capable than they describe and they do not use all his abilities. Secondly, reality is so diverse and colorful and still they do not bother to study it and find more creative solutions for their patients.

<u>The second approach is the approach of the scholastic culture. This approach stands for bypasses.</u> When we use a bypass we bypass the symptom or the "problematic" element and move determinedly forward towards a friendly goal while making efforts and concentrating. And to everybody's bewilderment, in most cases the symptom disappears. The new experience, which develops ability, replaces the symptom; enjoyment replaces fear.

Let's take for example an artist who wants to perform for a live audience, but suffers from stage fear and refers to psychological therapy. If he finds a nice psychologist, he will feel relaxed and secured during the sessions but he will still feel terrible before going on stage. On the other hand, if he forces himself to perform time and time again for anybody who is willing to watch him, and gradually expands his audience, he will learn eventually to enjoy performing for people. It is not enough to know how to sing and play; one should also have the ability to refer to other people, to perform for them, to serve them and to provide enjoyment. A persistent person will find out that the initial anxiety is replaced by a sense of pleasant excitement before going on stage. When such a person becomes a professional he will find out that he is at his best in front of an audience.

Another example is a case in which change is achieved by acting against our current feelings. A motorcycle rider who experienced a road accident attempts to ride his motorcycle again. He drives slowly with his eyes almost shut and his body shivers from anxiety. He believes that if he surrenders to anxiety it will make him give in the riding. He decides to resist his instincts, rides to the highway, turns the gas handle and reaches a speed of 120 kilometer per hour. A minute later, anxiety becomes almost unbearable, and then, all of the sudden, it is gone.

Another person feels that he is scared of walking by the cemetery alone at night. He decides that he is not going to be intimidated by ghosts and demons. He walks into a cemetery alone in the middle of the night, smokes a cigarette on one of the gravestones, pees just to spite and leaves. Another fear is knocked-out.

Another example: in therapeutic culture a person wakes up in the morning, attentive to his feelings, and feels a profound distress on the verge of minor depression. He does not feel like going out of bed and his thoughts are focused on the gloomy feelings. Injustice, insults, angers, deprivation, worries that are always there. Until noontime he becomes heavier and by evening he is totally depressed. In scholastic culture we do not obey these kinds of feelings. True, I do not expect a person who feels bad to wake up enthusiastically, but I surely expect him to do a more friendly deed and not to lie still and wait for his feelings to go away. A person is capable of concentrating real hard and finding something he is capable of doing, something more worthwhile than lying in bed. He could go to the beach, or trim bushes, or dig or do anything else which is simple and available. He will find out that perhaps it did not make him a happy person, but he certainly feels better than he felt when he woke up. And from this point, it is easier to move forward and add more and more activities that encourage him until he gets back to his old self. We bypass the feeling and instead of dwelling on it, we focus on other things.

If he keeps shaping his days he will start enjoying the things he does – enjoying his life in general and only a major disaster might cause him to suffer for a while.

The friendly "working instrument" can be used to better organize one's time. What can be done and what should be done. Not just to kill time but to combine fascinating activities in our daily routine. In Friendship School this approach is highly successful. It is especially efficient for people who are addicted to things they consider unfriendly but find it hard to get rid of. For instance, kicking the habit of heavy eating. The common approach is that a diet is needed. It is not that difficult to lose some kilograms, even many kilograms, but it is difficult to change one's eating habits and keeping one's weight for long periods of time. Most people who went on a diet eventually go back to their old eating habits. In such cases, I do not believe in self-restraint. It only increases the awareness of food and the person remains occupied with the subject instead of minimizing its importance. Moreover, people tend to rebel when they need to give in something they are addicted to and it might even cause them to become more addictive. Self-restraint may turn to an outbreak of eating mania. Thus, I suggest a bypass – filling the time with interesting, fascinating activities and by doing so developing gratifications that compete with the immediate gratifications derived from food. In other words, through the bypass we no longer deal with self-restraint and prevention of joy, but we move forward towards more sophisticated enjoyments. In such a case **the ending of the addiction is the by-product of discovering a better ability**. For instance, a person who has learnt to play bridge will find out that he is no longer addicted to poker and he did not even have to restrain himself. In fact, he will discover that he enjoys bridge better and even becomes addicted to this new game.

In case of a heavy addiction, another, not negative, addiction should be developed. For instance, exercising a lot on a daily basis until it becomes an addiction. Then we have a tool that can defeat another heavy addiction such as addiction to drugs or alcohol. If you play bridge all the time, until you become addicted to it, you can easily defeat an addiction to gambling.

There is another course for bypassing symptoms. Making a distinction between being alone and not being alone. Dwelling on the symptoms is something you do alone. But when you are not alone, there is a factor that forces you to focus on it. For example, a little boy, an important client or an audience you are supposed to entertain keep you company. When you are focused on referring to other people you forget about yourself and rest from your symptoms. In my case, for example, meeting a client makes me forget hunger, thirst and various pains as if the world does not exist and I do not exist.

(A comment regarding common approaches in culture that have varied titles: New Age, Mysticism, the Secret and the like. If you really intend to believe and desire something. it will eventually happen. I find these approaches captivating since they provide an illusion that there is no need to make changes in reality, and that a certain ritual activity, such as prayer, is sufficient.and can replace the hard work of developing abilities. I have examined many approaches and found out that producing ability provides a reliable solution and that is the reason I recommend it. The realistic approach also contains elements which are easy to achieve and one should start with them. Taking a motorcycle riding lesson, juggling three oranges, playing the harmonica etc. We can not run away from long-term investments if we want to learn how to play the violin or become a medicine etc). See: "Management," "Production."

Causality

Analytical thinkers believe that there is a relationship between cause and effect. Thus, when one comes across a problem, he must investigate and find the cause of it. This approach has caused, in my opinion, tremendous damage to a multitude of patients. Searching for a hidden cause, deep in the sub-consciousness, has led to a waste of time and money at the expense of the patients' lives and made them dwell on the problems. It has been very effective as far as the gurus of psychology are concerned since they knew how to explain the secrets of sub-consciousness to their obedient patients. Analytical thinking is of course a great tool which helps us solve many problems in the universe. It is especially essential for **technological products**. A decent plumber who was called after an apartment was flooded, must examine the pipes and discover where the leak is. Knowing the problem immediately leads to its solution. The same goes for an electrical system. In case of a failure we look for the cause and immediately know what needs to be fixed.

Friendly thinking which refers to human beings rather than to appliances assumes that numerous variables take part in an event to the extent that it is almost impossible to expose and discover all of the components. And even if it were possible, it is such a hassle that takes up much time and money at the expense of the patient, and most importantly, this knowledge will not contribute to the production of change.

Abilities and scholastic culture grant us freedom of choice. Among other things we have the freedom to decide what to take from our past and what to leave behind. Freedom is not unlimited. We are burdened with **genetic predispositions** that were passed to us from prior generations. And there is no doubt that experiences from early childhood have a great impact on our lives. As our mother tongue is rooted in our brain more than any other language we learn. As a result, our abilities are limited. I cannot become taller. Thus, I will not be able to become a professional basketball player. I can compensate for my height with other capabilities related to basketball. It is true, but why should I insist on developing these abilities instead of promoting more easily achieved capabilities which can lead me to more suitable destinations?

People have an amazing learning ability more than any other animal on the face of the earth. We should use this ability and realize our freedom of choice as much as possible. If we have a predisposition to be overweight, we should activate a special operating system which can minimize the effect of genetics. If we immigrate to a new country we should especially focus on learning the local language until it pushes our mother tongue aside. We should operate a system of special **compensation** for past shortcomings. We should rebel against whatever we can in order to realize the freedom of choice that was given to us.

Compensation

Luck is an important part of life. Where we were born, whom we were born to, what period we are born into, in which part of the world, etc. We develop with a certain amount of cultural and genetical data. There is no use comparing ourselves to others who have abilities we do not have. That is a fact. We are not equal. I suggest referring to the differences between ourselves and others as a decree, like immigration to a new country. A person who immigrates to another country and culture must make special efforts in order to master a language and a culture which are already familiar to the old residents. A person who is not committed to this effort is doomed to remain in a cultural enclave. If we make the move easier for the person, he will achieve less. It is similar to children who are diagnosed as suffering from learning disabilities and are entitled to various bonuses and perks. They usually achieve less than the others. The ones who make tremendous efforts achieve much more. Some students become better than their teachers.

Thus, in Friendship School, a person who has a certain development bug should not discuss it endlessly. If such a person is determined to produce change, he will simply have to work much harder than others. He must **compensate** for his neglected area with intensive efforts.

For instance, a forty-five year old bachelor who has never been in a serious relationship still has a chance to produce change in his life. The condition is that he must be committed to doing difficult homework, which he might even find crazy, until he learns to be a friend and a spouse. A person who invests only small efforts will progress a little, gradually, but will not succeed in making a change in his identity. He comes to see me from time to time, with his spouse, exhausted from work, choked and hostile, clenches his muscles as if he has just walked half a marathon and his entire being wishes to get rid of the woman and go back to his previous life. I often use the metaphor of a pilot's ejection seat. A person who is not used to the presence of a spouse and children sometimes desires a button that will eject him to another place in a second, or alternatively, eject the other people.

I allow him short periods of rest but do not allow rejection or prolonged rest. I tell him he will rest when he has family and children. Not a moment sooner. Because, if he rests now, as he feels like doing, he might not get to a stage of starting a family and will probably make do with much less.

Psychotherapy which is based on merely support and empathy is damaging. It eliminates the chance of producing change. I would leave the support to people who suffer from terminal diseases, to bring them human comfort.

Concentration

A molecule of ability which is essential both for learning and for enjoyment.

We may activate this ability in a certain domain and not in other domains. For example, sometimes teachers complain that a child has difficulties in concentration and that is not true. The child can be fascinated for hours by a computer game, while at school he chooses not to concentrate on the lesson either because he is not interested in it, or because he allows himself not to make an effort. Concentration is an important component for a person who wishes to join the scholastic culture which produces friendly changes.

When we learn new things, the doing requires a high level of concentration before it becomes an automatic act which does not require investment of energy. A child who wants to learn how to read, for instance, cannot just go over the black marks. If he does not concentrate on whatever he sees, combine the letters into words and the words into sentences, he will not acquire reading skills.

It is not possible to undergo profound emotional change without the ability to concentrate. A person who lacks the essential tools for acquiring new abilities, such as concentration, keeps reinforcing the old, predictable language and the diagnosis which have been planted in his brain. He locks himself within his limitations and misses the opportunity to increase his ability and produce change. **This molecule of ability is perhaps the most important one** <u>in scholastic</u>

culture. You should sharpen it. It enables creation of bypasses over the automatic mechanisms in the brain. It enables us to decide and to choose the things we should refer to. It facilitates freedom of choice. And of course, it is the basis of the superb entertaining quality related to our ability to enjoy ourselves. As you probably know, a person needs to concentrate in order to enjoy. Sexual intercourse in itself or tickets to a concert do not guarantee pleasure. Only concentration and listening produce maximal enjoyment.

This is the difference between the approach of Friendship School and most of the psycho-dynamic approaches. From the start a person has a certain ability to concentrate on a certain task, such as reading, for a while. Let's assume that at the moment your ability is not that great and you need to make an effort in order to concentrate. You manage to read five lines and then you get too tired and your consciousness drifts away. According to most approaches you should pay attention to the source of distraction, follow it and even write it down. You need to understand where it comes from, what is bothering you etc. In the meantime your reading ability remains stuck at the same place. In Friendship School, the minute you notice that you lost your concentration on the lines you are reading, you bring yourself back to it. The content of the distraction is totally insignificant. You read another five lines, and once again, your thoughts drift away. You bring yourself back to the relevant stimulus, which is reading, at once. You read another five lines, which constitute your current concentration ability, or even reread the previous lines in order to plant them better in your brain, until you feel you cannot go further. Take a break. A few hours later, go back to the task of concentrating on the lines. Within a few days you will discover that your reading ability has improved tremendously. The minute you fix your eyes on the print, you do not let go and read whole pages before you feel the need to rest. Now you do not need to rest every five lines but only after reading five pages. You should be persistent in promoting your ability and you will discover that you can read a whole book at once easily and enjoyably. This is also a critical junction for producing change.

See: "Junction of Opportunities."

Of course you can practice your concentration also by listening to classical music until you know the piece by heart.

Sharpening the ability of deciding what you should concentrate on resembles vision focus. The minute you fix your eyes on an object, it seems clear. All other objects within the field of vision seem vague and objects which are beyond the field of vision are not seen at all. You decide to turn your head and focus on a different object and by doing so your whole field of vision changes. **Thus, one should not even bother to remove a certain object. It is sufficient to focus on something.** Anything else either goes away or disappears altogether as a result of our concentration.

Reliable concentration ability enables us to reach conclusions about our priorities. When we concentrate well on all our occupations we have a reliable tool for comparing the different occupations and identifying which ones better reflect us, which ones are most enjoyable. Without this ability, conclusions do not mean much, for we do not have an adequate tool for reaching conclusions.

Constraint

Tasks, obligations, and things we are forced to do.

At one extreme we will find people who live their lives handcuffed, sometimes to the extent that they repress and eliminate all sense of desire. They do not enjoy freedom of choice. They can only chose between a greater obligation and a smaller one. For instance, your mother is sick and your aunt is sick – you must first take care of your mother. Or, if you are religious, for a matter of life and death the Sabbath can be broken, but you could not possibly imagine going hiking with your family on Sabbath. On weekdays you are committed to your job and your studies and on Sabbath you are committed to praying and to dictated rest.

Many of us have not yet sharpened their tools of choice and screening and for them, identity issues and daily decisions which need to be considered time and time again are an unbearable burden. They prefer settings in which all answers are given in advance. These people escape from freedom to rigorous settings such as religion, army, high-tech and the like. They are busy up to their necks. Next to them we will find people who are constantly busy with nuisances - worries in general and health worries in particular. The nature of the worries is not important. What is important is the level of their awkwardness. It could be a compulsive pursuit of tidiness and cleanliness or of various "errands," waiting in line in different waiting rooms, telephone conversations and correspondence with different authorities' officials. They believe they would have preferred to have fun and enjoy themselves if a certain unfortunate business had not been forced upon them. But they cannot break loose. When they finish dealing with a certain concern, a new concern suddenly appears. The awkwardness starts when one does not distinguish between a constraint to run to the hospital with a kid who has broken his leg and a "constraint" to fill in various forms and run from clerk to clerk in order to get a $25 carfare refund. The latter is about a sense of duty and not a constraint forced upon us.

Treating and healing obsessive compulsiveness is done through pleasure: learning to concentrate on and persist in different actions until the ability to enjoy is created. An individual who has learning difficulties needs a medication. He will not learn to enjoy life but the medication will lighten the burden on his shoulders.

For your information, although it may be seen as a contradiction, the people who are able to meet their obligations and deal with constraints are equipped with whatever is necessary in order to produce changes through learning and persistence. For instance, when such a person is asked to learn something new, or when a difficult change is needed, he will have a clear advantage over many adults who have already become fixated, move only when they "feel like it" and avoid efforts.

Thus, in Friendship School, we recommend starting the process of change as a constraint until change becomes a fulfilling, exciting part of our identity. Starting the change is done through homework. In order to prevent misunderstandings, little children do not need constraints in order to learn. They are equipped with the best learning tools and learn all the time by way of amusement. And if a certain change is required, all they need is an adult who knows how to have fun with them, and he could easily bring about the change. But an adult who has already become fixated and has fixed habits should not wait until he feels the urge for a change. He should start the change arbitrarily.

See "Management."

Crude Rejection

An automatic reaction to whatever we are exposed to that does not fit our regular abilities.

Crude rejection is an automatic reaction, a predictable reaction to things that do not suit our regular abilities. There are many manifestations of the awkwardness of this reaction. The most common manifestation is "no." A person is exposed to a certain proposal and says "no," often without even listening to the nature of the proposal: "I don't have time," "I don't have money," "I don't feel like it" etc. These people do not make a distinction between "I don't have money to go to the movies with a friend " and "I don't have money to go on a journey around the world on a fancy yacht. ; they do not make a distinction between the mountain and the molehill and react in a similar way to two completely different things. Or, in other words, the awkwardness is sometimes expressed by the fact that the reaction to a certain thing we cannot possibly do at a certain time also eliminates the things we can do. For instance, a young mother who works very hard taking care of her baby might fall ill: when she feels bad someone else takes care of the baby since there is no alternative; but the illness also prevents her from doing other things she could do. A more sophisticated mother would not need a **crude means** such as illness in order to rest a little bit, but would allow herself various intermissions. From time to time she would find a reliable person to take care of her baby, and would make the time to go shopping, take a walk, go out or rest.

Another version of this reaction is crude diagnosis such as "this is difficult!" with an exclamation mark instead of "I find it difficult right now." For example, when someone makes crude diagnosis such as "mathematics is a difficult subject," it is as if the diagnosis becomes a solid fact and there are no more negotiations. This important point should be clarified. When a person knows he cannot be taller he does not aspire to become a basketball player and does not try to change it. Some people do not make a distinction between the **sense** of inability and real inability and believe that whatever they feel reflects the reality, meaning that if they encounter difficulties they believe it is difficult and they do not try to change it. Sometimes such a person makes certain gestures of change and tells himself and others - I have tried and did not succeed – and reaches the conclusion that it is, indeed, unchangeable and by doing so he reinforces the diagnosis planted in his mind and eliminates the chance of making a change. This is very common "brain damage" which locks the person in a dungeon of his automatic programming. Many people repeat the school year time and time again as if the clock has stopped.

However, in scholastic culture there is a **more accurate perception** of the relation between current ability and future possibilities. Namely, a person realizes he has a difficulty in mathematics since he is not familiar with the subject, and not because it is a difficult subject in particular. So there is a chance that if he decides to proceed and learn mathematics, and do it gradually and persistently, he will find out that his ability increases and the things that were difficult for him in the beginning become easy. The opposite of a crude rejection is an attempt to be accurate! That is the maximal diminution according to which we will do exactly what we can do. No more, no less.

Another common manifestation of crude rejection is **inciting**: when you think of an idea – and immediately put it off through a contradicting idea. Instead of placing the ideas side by side, analyzing them thoroughly, and then making a friendly decision – diminishing the idea at the first place. This is common amongst supposedly "judgmental" people, who always rush into finding disadvantages (nothing is perfect!) and use them in order to disqualify everything. This is how they destroy the pluses through the minuses and ruin the good and the bad. A common example of this type of crude rejection can be found amongst chronic singles who find disadvantages in every potential partner and by doing so miss any possible enjoyment. <u>Friendly thinking</u> and scholastic culture are about scanning the scenery of opportunities, noticing a few "packages" of stimulations, each containing minuses and pluses, comparing them – and choosing a favorite one, disadvantages included.

The role of such crude rejection means is to minimize the world at once and adjust it to our current reservoir of abilities. This is an automatic mechanism whose role is to maintain the status quo and to prevent change as much as possible, including changes which a person thinks he might be interested in. Various symptoms demonstrate that, from blowups to various maladies, fears and anxieties. I do not make a distinction between a migraine and falling in love, when dealing with both interrupts the concentration in whatever is more relevant to a person's life. The nature of the symptom is irrelevant; there is no difference if the barrier placed by the person between himself and the opportunity is made of migraine, falling in love or compulsive thoughts. The reason a person chooses to reject in a certain way while his friend rejects in another way is insignificant. Everybody develops or adapts rejections which are suitable for them.

Sometimes I will refer to the **intensity** of the side effects of the process of change and suggest taking them into account. I will do that when a person reacts real awkwardly in a way that jeopardizes his life. We must make a distinction between side effects such as infections, sore throat, fever, itches and severe road accidents. We will bypass moderate symptoms and move forward till they disappear on their own. In case severe symptoms appear it is advisable to examine how essential the change is for realizing the person's identity. We might even want to give up the change. In other words, we might prefer that the person remains where he is, safe and sound, to a situation that he keeps changing while jeopardizing his health and his life.

It should be noted that when the rejections are directed towards the guide and the client is not able to bypass them, he might neutralize the accompaniment of the guide who tries to help him to bypass the means of the rejection and to mediate between him and the opportunity to change.

Thus, a crude rejection is whatever a person puts between himself and the relevant stimulus. In therapeutic culture, it seems that people deal with irrelevant things, namely, "problems," and get stuck in the same place. In scholastic culture, we refer to symptoms as side effects, which are predictable during the first stages of change or the learning process; like calluses on hands which are not used to hard work, or excitement on the verge of anxiety in light of an unusual event. In scholastic culture we focus on the relevant stimulus – namely, on whatever promotes us further. Indeed, as aforementioned, if we do not linger on the symptoms, but keep learning and experiencing patiently and gradually, ability increases, the symptoms vanish and instead we experience pleasure originated from realizing our ability. **When we obey the symptom and act according to it, it becomes a rejection means**; and when we bypass the symptom, focus intensively on the difficult things, and when we are determined to move forwards in spite of the symptoms, ability continues to develop and the symptoms disappear, without having to spend unnecessary energy on them. For instance, if a woman who has intercourse experiences pain during penetration, and her reaction is to obey the pain and prevent it by avoiding sexual intercourse – she adapts a crude rejection means: an illness called "vaginismus." On the other hand, if she continues to focus on her partner, and goes to bed with him frequently, but does not burden herself with impossible missions all at once, but focuses on caressing, then mutual caressing and adds more and more components to the intimate encounter, the pains might be replaced by enjoyment. [In parenthesis: The insight described above was the main reason I quitted the heaven of belonging to the prevalent psychology culture. Therapists who spend many hours listening to descriptions of the patient's symptoms and enable him to describe what he feels and senses over and over again, encourage him to remain with the same means of rejection. When the patient describes his senses of inability time and time again, the same senses are fixated in his brain as an unchangeable fact. That misses the mark terribly and it means his potential abilities will not be realized. Even if a certain change is created, it seems that his diagnosis as the one with the problem limits the potential change. He will achieve very little, very slowly when he could have achieved much more faster and more easily if only he had been committed to do what he **can**, instead of what he senses. Quite a few families came apart with the "help" of professionals who listened emphatically to her descriptions of him and his descriptions of her; listening that supposedly turned the feelings into facts. I do not intend to claim that people must stay together forever. Sometimes couples face unbridgeable gaps, and they are better off with worthier partners. A move that might include significant change, that might even justify the high cost of divorce, but, in most cases, people destroy whatever they have built so far in exchange for much less than what they had. Usually, the woman becomes a single parent with limited connection to men, and the man is back at the meat market of blind dates and partial relationships. I assume people's emotions are based on their past experiences. People who bother to adapt abilities which they did not have in the past will find out soon enough that they have new feelings that were not felt in the past. Such a person learns how to love things he did not love before, and love less the things he was addicted to in the past since his world is now much wider. But we should not criticize the psychologists who earn their living from people who are willing to pay great sums of money to a person who is willing to listen or willing to pretend he is listening. In Friendship School we will offer these people to find a listener for free amongst neighbors and friends, and we will listen to them when they have the ability to contribute. If, for instance, a patient is a history expert, we will listen to him as much as he wants and we will benefit from it]. Crude rejection severely disrupts learning processes. As long as a person keeps rejecting whatever he is not familiar with, he will not change. He is a <u>learning decliner</u>. Using crude rejection means harms the person's identity since he becomes much more limited than he could have been. It also harms the person's reality perception, since reality is perceived only by his judgmental eyes that look at it through a narrow slit and miss the diversified scenery which contains many friendly paths.

As aforementioned, crude rejection means are designed to limit our world and adjust it to the reservoir of existing abilities so that we will not have to learn and change. Thus, we must recruit our full ability and force in the face of this reflex. We must use every sophisticated, cunning tool in order to destroy the crude rejection means or at least to bypass and neutralize it.

Nevertheless, rejection is sometimes caused due to our inability to distinct between the things we really cannot do at a certain point, and the things we can do. **How can we make a distinction between inability and the sense of inability?** If we wish to find out about our real limitations, we will ask ourselves whether in the face of a real threat we would avoid the act and say that "it cannot be done." We cannot possibly add another meter to our height, not even in the face of such a threat; but perhaps we would be able to run faster. In most cases we are not confronted by circumstances which force us to realize our maximal abilities. In order to start a change, we should, therefore, use our imagination – we should imagine a threat hanging over our head, and act. This is, no doubt, the concept which is the most difficult to understand. Friendly attitude towards ourselves and the reality often means seeing reality in a new way we are not used to and to act, from time to time, contrary to the way we sense, feel and think. Obviously, it is not that easy. It is not easy to identify crude rejection, and even if we do identify it, it is not easy to bypass it. Strict thinking discipline is required in order to realize that in most cases the strong emotional reaction is in fact against **strong stimulations**. For instance, you cannot stand your spouse not because you think he is no good, but because he is much more than you can love or contain. It is like ultra-Orthodox people who react with disgust and hostility to a sexy woman who comes to their neighborhood. If you ask them why they feel this way, they will say that the woman is despicable, but people with a greater realm of understanding would easily notice that religious people who watch TV, go to the beach in the summer, watch movies and read books besides the Holy Scriptures do not respond with a sense of rejection. On the contrary, they would feel aroused. The first group is not even allowed to **have** emotions, which are essentially perceived as forbidden.

Similarly, a mother who explodes over the fact that her daughter is sleeping peacefully at noon is actually aroused, or "jealous," of her daughter's ability to idle while she is forced to clean, tidy and work as hard as an ant. If, for example she takes a crash course in "idleness,," she will not feel the same way towards her daughter.

An additional comment or even a clarification regarding the **intensity** of this violent reaction: an interesting point – why do the Orthodox hate the Reformists more than they hate the Gentiles? Since the Gentiles do not constitute a stimulus or a threat for that matter as a monkey on a tree does not encourage you to be like it. However, a friend at the Yeshiva becomes more and more secular, he triggers much rejection and hostility since he constitutes a stimulation. His friends face someone who allows himself something they prevent from themselves – freedom. It is not easy for them to be around someone who used to be like them and is able to free himself from the fear of God. Similarly, a person who shows signs of becoming a believer will cause some of his friends to react with disgust, contempt and assault. Those who react this way probably wish they could also rest from the burden of freedom and the need to constantly choose and decide and become part of a culture that contains many more exclamation marks than question marks.

Here, as far as I know, lays the insight regarding the cause of violent reactions in society. I prefer this insight since it leads to friendly solutions. Not moral education but a commitment of the educational system to teach abilities necessary for living with people who are different from us.

Is everybody who wishes to leave his spouse reacting with crude rejection? Not necessarily. So **how can we make the distinction between crude rejection and friendly and free choice?**

This is an open-ended question. One clear sign is the **intensity of hatred**. A woman who wishes to divorce her husband because she no longer benefits from the relationship, because the gaps are increasing and she does not enjoy the relationship anymore, but does not hate her husband – this may be an example of free choice. Another clear sign is: a person refuses an offer because he **has** something better may be an example of screening. The waiving is the result of selecting a different option. For example, when a pupil enters the fifth grade, he no longer studies in the fourth grade. But when someone who does not have a girlfriend rejects the opportunity to meet a girl, it is considered a crude rejection and it does not matter how he convinced himself that he is better off not meeting her. Another example is an unemployed person who refuses to work because the salary is not high enough. He remains unemployed and weakens himself. In the future he will have to make extra efforts in order to rejoin the labour market. It is better for him to accept the job, and in the future, when he finds a more interesting and rewarding job, he will be able to quit the previous one.

Ability, and only ability, grants the right to choose. When a person is capable of A and is also capable of B, the word "preference" might mean something, when he prefers something to the other. When a person lacks ability – he cannot possibly prefer or choose.

Culture Pocket

People who choose to belong to a group which separates itself from the rest of the world and live in a kind of social ghetto characterized by a certain culture.

There are many different examples of culture pockets: a homogeneous religious group, which separates itself from the rest of society, such as a mystic cult, an Indian ashram, or ultra-Orthodox Jews who only concentrate on learning the Torah in a closed environment; immigrants who live in a community whose members come only from a certain country and do not learn the language or culture of the new country; career people who devote all their time to their work; people who suffer from chronic depression and are shut in their house; criminals who feel more at home in prison than in their own house.

Children who are born into a culture pocket are shaped in the spirit of their limited environment. The people who have interests in this culture pocket hope that since the children are never exposed to the rest of the world, they will reject everything which does not suit their culture even when they are grown-ups.

In trampled culture, an encounter of two culture pockets creates negative conflicts that sometimes become violent; in scholastic culture encounters broaden the horizons of the members of the two groups and enrich them. Thus, for instance, we will observe with pleasure and interest an ultra-Orthodox, Moroccan, Russian or secular wedding.

See: "Blocking."

Days' content

Everything we do during the day.

The Days' content is a working tool. In order to know the kind of homework we should do, we must be aware of the way we build our schedule. It is not about planning one special day, but a consecutive series of days, including weekends. The days' content includes the activities we do during the day and the people we spend our time with. When we look at the day that has passed, we should examine to what extent we did what is appropriate for us or how much of our time was devoted to unnecessary activities. Who are the people who contribute to us and who are the people who just waste our time? Do we pass the time passively waiting for events to take place, or are we in control of our time? It is important for us to know that we are the designers of our days' content and we are able to change it. Some people invest only in a single domain at a given period since they believe that they should not overburden themselves. That is a common mistake. "First I finish my studies and then I will start to work, and only when I have enough time and money I will start a family."

This kind of thinking leads the person to build a narrow, thin identity and he will not achieve much, if at all. In Friendship School we will impose more burdens in order to build the skills that enable a student to study, work in temporary jobs, develop relationships, etc. You can imagine a timetable, similar to what you had in school, but instead of English, literature and arithmetic, we plant the subjects which are relevant to a student in Friendship School.

This is a personal timetable. It includes work, studies, relationship, parenthood, hobbies and anything else we agree on.

The days' content is a tool which enables us to learn about ourselves and from time to time to do a kind of bookkeeping or learn lessons that will be applied afterwards. Designing the next days is a great tool for shaping our identity and start up productions which improve our self-expression and our satisfaction with our life.

See: "Management," "Production," "Homework."

Dealing with "Problems"

What can be done after you have established an identity of a person with a problem?

Don't be wise after the event.

Most problems are easily avoidable through friendly growth and educational processes. We should adapt a culture that nourishes ability and does not castrate and oppress. For instance, we should first let a child experience preparing a salad and only afterwards, when his ability is improved, we should teach him how to tidy up the mess in the kitchen. In a culture that takes the child into account the parents do not quarrel or swear in front of the child and at the same time this type of culture nourishes the child's ability to be considerate towards others.

The most important thing is to avoid diagnostic processes of children as these might be lethal. In these diagnostic processes every insignificant symptom is granted a title. "Lack of coordination," "Violent," "ADHD" and so forth. It is easier to produce change before attaching the awkward derogatory nickname. Obviously, in order to be born in a friendly environment one should be lucky and not all of us are. Thus, we should adapt tools which will help us to bypass problems and blockings and develop our identity.

Let's discuss a common diagnosis such as:

"Low Self Image"

I put the title in inverted commas since I refuse to define a person according to such a judgment. When this judgment is repeated over and over again it becomes a fact and not merely an assessment. As no one expects a tree to start walking, as a result of the judgmental facts, no one expects a change. That is what I call "brain damage." Positive judgments are usually awkward as well. One should make an effort and be accurate when referring to abilities. "He is a genius" is a common judgment amongst mothers. In most cases it is means that the child has certain high-quality ability and that the mother is short-sighted. Leonardo da Vinci might have been a genius. How many are like him? "My wife is a superb cook" (this is usually a spouse's enthusiastic assessment alongside common assessments such as "does not do anything" if the wife is a housewife). Well, that might be a pretty accurate assessment, when referring to a professional chef who spends most of her time cooking. "My wife baked a cake" – is a fact. "My wife cooks a lot" – is also a fact if she spends much of her time cooking and so forth.

If so, discussing low self image, detailed descriptions of the sense of humiliation and descriptions of castrating experiences do not contribute to change. They spread within the soul as a plague and infect domains of abilities with a sense of helplessness. Moreover, dwelling on past and searching for the origin of our tendency to undermine ourselves do not add confidence at all. How important is the fact that our mother undermined our father in the distant past or that we have been oppressed and castrated? Now, when you are a grownup, no one can influence you that way. If you feel today the same as you felt as a little child it means you have repressed your ability to grow and develop. On the other hand, when we invest in learning and experiencing, our ability develops and we become experts. We would probably feel confident in the specific domain we have chosen. Our fingers flutter on the piano keys and we do not need to look at the notes; we know for certain who wrote *War and Peace*; we are able to fix electrical appliances at home. More action, less talk. Emotions will not change unless real action takes place. People who have specialized in a single field would feel confident in this narrow domain, but beyond it they would feel a lack of confidence and deep perplexity. On the other hand, people who constantly promote numerous abilities in various domains will find out soon enough that they become confident, almost arrogant. Realizing they have the ability to learn becomes a major part of their identity. Every additional proficiency contributes to our confidence as long as the new ability was not programmed in us in the past. A person who knows how to read and reads another book does not surprise anyone, but when a person who is afraid of water learns to swim it means that he has experienced the ability to learn that can also be reflected in learning how to juggle balls, ride a bicycle hands-free, ride a rollercoaster and the like.

Soon he realizes that once he is committed to a new domain, makes efforts and invest resources, he will become an expert in this new field as well. Meeting capable people who once made him feel pitiable and castrated in comparison, will become an interesting stimulation. A stimulation to nurture more and more capabilities. Obviously, my description of the contents of one of the common symptoms which become an awkward diagnosis is random. I could have chosen to write in detail about anxiety, guilt, depression and so forth. Instead of referring to the symptoms, we should refer to people's abilities which can serve as the basis for change. Let us examine another example, "**depression.**" First we should examine the things that the person does on a daily basis. Let's take for example a young man who does not have a female friend or regular sex life. A person who neglects such an important area cannot possibly feel good about himself. Even if we presume he has a reason to do so – his lover has abandoned him – it is obvious that as he dwells on the abandonment and the pain, he becomes more and more addicted to depression. Indeed, many people waste years doing just that. In <u>friendly thinking</u> **the main reason for depression is that a person allows himself not to do what he is capable of doing**. Each one of us **must** express his abilities. The deserted young man must force himself to relate to one of the other women who are available and he will not suffer any longer. If he is so "heavy" and he finds it difficult to entertain a female friend, he should experience another positive immediate relief such as sports. By doing so he will experience a movement forward and can use this improvement to pursue more significant productions.

Sometimes, when people do not succeed in producing such friendly actions, it is possible to take antidepressant medication for a while in order to be able to go back to the appropriate activities.

"Quarrels"

A common rejection means amongst people who have not succeeded in finding something more interesting to do together. They are not able to contain each other and they need a rest from each other. The quarrel serves as an awkward break from couplehood. They do not know how to rest from each other through more sophisticated, civilized means. For instance, the man is resting in one room and the woman is reading in another. Indeed, they are not spending time together, but they are not spending their time quarreling. From this point it is very easy to start enjoying each other, while people who are used to quarrels spend a great deal of energy on forbearance and reconciliation before they can do pleasant things together.

I refer to quarrels as a cultural disability. When people allow themselves to spend time together without taking into account the fact that they are not alone they allow themselves to burden other people, for instance, when a person picks his nose during a family dinner.

When two spouses are interested in making a change and cooperate, it is easy to produce it. First, we do not dwell on the contents of the quarrels since it would further enforce the fixation. For a period of a few weeks they are not allowed to be with each other without planning the time in advance. Since at the beginning they are not capable of loving each other and enjoying each other, the proximity and friction constitute a negative stimulation and a quarrel breaks out. Later, their mutual fields of interest expand until the entertaining quality becomes better. At this point, in most cases when people are able to choose between an appropriate pastime and a quarrel, they prefer the pastime. Obviously, part of their homework is to work out a lot, together if possible, and in addition to add another position or two to their sex life.

It is more complicated to produce change when only one of the spouses makes an effort. This spouse must break off contact as long as the relationship remains negative. He is making a declaration that it is not possible to be with him and be unpleasant at the same time. Sometimes, it suffices to make the change. But, sometimes the other spouse enjoys the estrangement. The dosage of togetherness suits his limitations. In this case, I will recommend the capable spouse to make up for the lack by finding a friendly connection outside of the relationship.

Delinquency

A person who is willing to deviate from the norm into places that are rejected by public opinion.

This term does not refer to unfriendly delinquency which is punishable by the state, but to actions that the delinquent could not even imagine himself doing prior to the change.

Delinquency is important. When we want to change we must be aware of the fact that change could make other people, especially from the group we were used to be part of, perceive us as "wrong." Thus, we should develop our skill of being delinquent and overpower numerous prohibitions which were part of our education. It is important to note that the term "delinquency" is meaningful only in the social context which it belongs to. For instance, driving a car on Saturday is considered a "felony" in a Jewish religious community. **"A delinquency course" is** especially **essential** for people who suffer from feelings of guilt and whose inhibitions prevent them from achieving desirable goals. They are not blocked to the extent that they do not have desires, on the contrary, they know what they want very well, but their brain is controlled by stern disciplinary processes. The course is also essential for good, well-bred people, in the negative sense of the word, namely, people who are obedient, content themselves with little, and accept their destiny. These people are not equipped with tools that enable change. Thus, they must first complete a sort of preparatory course that includes acts which contradict their initial programming.

For instance, an aging bachelor really wants to find a spouse and start a family. It is not such a difficult task. He starts dating women from his social circle or dates available women who are part of the Friendship School. However, during weekdays he works at a bakery mostly during evenings and nights. It was not so bad if he could at least compensate for that during the weekends. But lately he has started to keep the Sabbath. So that it is impossible to assist him with all the limitations he puts upon himself. He must either make schedule changes at work, or agree to violate the Sabbath.

Another example is of a mother who wants to go out instead of preparing a meal for her adolescent children. She finds it very difficult to do something which contradicts the behavior that she perceives as suitable for a mother. Another mother has a son who yells at her and kicks her from time to time and she finds it difficult to react. An hour after the outbreak she even buys him ice-cream on demand. A demand, not a request. I tell her: "Leave him with his grandmother for an hour and take a break." She says: "No, no I can't do that; he will have separation anxiety, it will damage his soul." It will damage him much more if he grows up knowing that he can hit whenever someone irritates him, and it might even cause him to get entangled with the law. But the mother is limited to act according to the motherhood program in her brain. If she does not take the preparatory course in delinquency she will be no good when it comes to educating her son.

Depression

Common, addictive pastime.
See: "Dealing with Problems."

Developing / Developmental Bug

Some refer to it as behavior pattern.
In order to identify a bug in development, one should scan a wide scenery which includes various states of aggregation and the person's abilities. An example of a severe bug is found in a person who is an adult but acts childishly. A person who still lives with his parents, does not work, does not study etc.

In most cases we will identify the bug in a person who has developed in certain channels quite impressively, but neglected growth in a particular channel. For instance, a single woman who has never had a spouse. She is forty years old and claims she is eager to start a family etc. She is an attractive woman and has magnificent abilities. If she believes that the issue is that she has only met defective men so far, then we have a problem. She must realize that if she has come so far without a spouse, it is not because there are not any men worthy of companionship, but because for some reason **she** does not know how to be a companion. Her bug is reflected in her choice of men with whom nothing can be developed and in the fact that she runs away from worthy men who want her. This is an **active** act which is meant to make sure that a stable, lasting relationship would never develop. She **chooses** men who fit her limited ability, men who are on the same page and who, like herself, have repeated the same school year time and time again. Surely, there are other men out there; men with first rate relationship abilities, but she does not find them interesting enough or they recognize her limited abilities and disqualify her as a partner. If she identifies a bug, she must do her homework – date men whom she does not like at first, and learn how to derive pleasure, interest and satisfaction from them. Totally "arbitrary" homework. In other words, not doing what she likes to do. Exactly as she would be forced to drive on the left side of the road if she were in London, regardless of her habits and convenience. I try to help my clients avoid paying tens of thousands of dollars and a few years of looking into their past and recollection of all their experiences so far. These are the practices of the traditional therapeutic model which is based on the assumption that the cause of the problem should be discovered and analyzed. As if knowing the reason will help them find a solution and produce change. I know for a fact that it does not contribute to change. On the contrary, in most cases the focus remains on the problem and it becomes fixated. I am happy enough when the clients recognize a certain bug in their growth mechanism and are willing, from that point on, to work in order to produce change. It requires a certain amount of reviewing their introspection throughout the years in order to identify repetitive patterns.

The bug is not diagnosed only by the fact that an individual has stopped doing something. For instance, stopped going to university, stopped painting or riding his bike. We must review what he was doing at that time. For example, learnt how to drive a car and even bought one. In this case he upgraded himself from a biker to a driver. His identity has changed. In the future he may return to his bike, in order to keep in shape or to spend time with his children. This is certainly not a bug. It is advisable to identify when someone is growing and developing, which means he is moving "forward" or "upward," from the less to the more, and when he is moving "sideways" or "backwards," from the more to the less.

Moreover, it should be noted that there are many channels of growth and development. A very young man who has not grown, built an identity as a spouse and has not started a family could become a skilled commander who is responsible for his soldiers. He will be the leader and the father in his unit.

In a scholastic culture, when there is no developmental bug, a constant leakage is possible. A leakage from one domain into other domains. Abilities which are channeled into all kinds of directions and possibilities. For instance, experience based on raising children could easily be channeled into command responsibility or management of employees.

It does not always develop linearly, sometimes there is skipping. For example, someone learns to be a mother and only afterwards becomes a spouse.

See "Causality."

Enforcement Tools

It is difficult to describe to what extent a certain bug in my clients' initial programming is change resistant. It is as if this bug has control over the person making sure that certain experiences repeat themselves. I try to convince my client to rebel against the force controlling his life, to defeat it altogether, or just to bypass it. I try to assist my client to take control over his own life.

Indeed, I keep trying but it does not always work.

The term "enforcement tools" expresses my helplessness. My tools are so limited when I sit on my couch trying to convince and influence someone to make a change. And I do not make do with sitting on the couch. Ever since I retired from traditional psychology, I have been doing everything I could possibly do, in order to promote change. Starting from housing the client in my home, in order to cut him off from undesirable influences, and expose him to a different culture, to house calls and all sorts of manipulations.

For sure, in Friendship School success rates are much higher compared with other methods, but much lower than what could have been achieved. More than once I get to know a client, review his capabilities, and talents and I am eager to help him realize his potential, while the client, in my opinion, contents himself with little. Here, the force of the bug in the initial programming is fully expressed and I feel helpless – I cannot defeat this bug when my client supports it.

The only tool at my disposal when I come across a learning decliner is to expel him from my school. I have decided not to earn a living by trying to help people who cannot be changed. On rare occasions, it does help. In most cases, it does not. This client will easily find a psychologist who will listen to him eagerly and not burden him with homework.

This is the reason I do not look for **the one with the problem**, but for **the person who has the ability** to produce change. In most cases, these are the parents or the spouses. If the spouse is wise and has the ability to influence, he is very significant to the one with the problem. He can assist in the process of change. I see it as an act of love.

When parents or spouses are also limited and helpless, or in case they have the ability but refuse to cooperate, there is nothing more I can do.

It should be mentioned, though, that I do not recommend starting with these enforcement tools. The best way of making a change is the pleasant way and by exposing the individual to enjoyable, entertaining cultural stimulations. But when an unfriendly pattern has already been fixated, we must prepare an alternative plan which includes influential tools which are not connected to the head, but to the "feet. For instance, if the child does not respond to friendly suggestions, he will find out it is not worthwhile, because he loses something. For example, his family goes on a trip without him since he did not bother to learn how to be considerate towards other people. Taking him to the trip, before he has changed, might spoil other people's enjoyment.

Entertaining Quality

The extent to which something we do entertains us.
In order to achieve maximal entertaining quality, we **must** concentrate on the activities with high attention level. If we do not concentrate on what we do, it is as if we swallow food without noticing the taste, as if we look but cannot see, hear but cannot listen. Only sufficient training will enable us to decide when to give good entertaining level and when to eliminate some things from our mind.

Activities which reflect our capabilities well have first rate entertaining quality. Some people enjoy their professions and hobbies. However, an addiction to negative factors such as pain, suffering or depression, could also be of high entertaining quality. In the past, psychologists used to say that some people "enjoy suffering." They talked about "masochistic pleasure." The word "pleasure" cannot be perceived in the context of suffering. Thus, I prefer to refer to "entertaining quality" or "recreation." Still, most people are expected to object to this approach. A negative activity is perceived by most people as something which is forced upon us by life circumstances beyond our control. But, I suggest making a distinction between events and habits. A negative feeling can indeed derive as an initial response to a certain traumatic event, but if it lasts for long, it becomes a habit, an addiction, recreation. I look at it from the cultural point of view. Some people spend their time with music, dancing and philosophy, while others focus on suffering, depression and idleness. The change occurs when such a person replaces the negative activities with other, friendly, cultural activities. With a little effort, almost anyone can find out how easy it is for him to feel negative feelings such as deprivation, offense, obsessive thoughts etc. It does no bore us. If we became addicted to a negative factor and we wish to stop the addiction, we must choose an **immediate relief which is not negative** – such as our favorite sport or an activity which fascinates us and is not related to pain and suffering. People who have not yet developed their identity and their ability channels will have to be extremely determined in order to establish their identity and get rid of the negative addiction.

Developing the ability to concentrate contributes a great deal to producing entertaining quality. The ones who have learnt to enjoy their actions and their surroundings live meaningful lives. Think of the difference between a person who sees the raising of his children as a constraint consisting of multiple burdensome tasks such as watching the children, feeding them, washing them, putting them to sleep, helping them with their homework, and all he wants is to complete the tasks and rest. And now think of someone who enjoys **spending time** with his children and perceives the tasks as additional elements and not as the focus. Think of the difference between someone who is married only "on paper" and someone who enjoys spending time with his spouse. Think of the difference between a person who works to support his family and a person who supports his family by focusing on his favorite hobby.

Friendly Thinking

Creating a section in the brain which bypasses automatic programming

This type of thinking enables people to produce positive changes and grow in <u>scholastic culture</u>. It also helps people to get rid of fixated thinking patterns which allow only minor changes. In friendly thinking we do not disqualify whatever is in our brain in advance, namely the emotional responses, but put it aside, and continue to scan the scenery of options without prior judgment. During the scan we ask ourselves, amongst other things, which option is best for us, what can we produce from it and whether it suits our capabilities. **The brain should actually be trained to control itself this way.**

We should scan the scenery without categorizing it immediately, without putting it in one of the already existing slots in our brain. We should not sort it out immediately as oranges are sorted into the right box, but leave it and continue the scan. By the way, a rush decision could be an immediate acceptance or immediate rejection. Perhaps in this case it will turn out to be a friendly decision, but it is not really so since it was not screened and selected after a thorough examination of capabilities and possibilities. This section in the brain which I refer to as the "landlord" restrains the horses in the brain that rush towards a certain goal, it continues the scan and rushes towards a goal which is selected only after the scan and the screening have been completed.

With the help of friendly thinking we will learn to identify whatever already exists in our brain: we will make a distinction between the predictable responses that are familiar to us, the opinions and judgments that are constantly uttered in a complex, changing reality and the things we are currently producing and are different from whatever was in our brain previously. We will try to air fixated opinions. These are the opinions we have always had despite of various, numerous variables which are piled in front of us. It is as if we put in front of the camera lens a picture which separates it from the reality in front of it. Obviously we should practice the act of selecting which is preferring one package deal over the others very often.

Nurturing the tool of friendly thinking resembles learning a new language. It is not easy, but it is worth it. The effort is most significant in the binding point of the change. In fact, the thing which is most likely to sabotage the decision to change is our enormous, misleading brain. Its prior programming attempts to protect itself from the change, qualify change as undesirable and knows how to "convince" us. A kind of a battle takes place against the "new management" and its attempt to take control over the whole organization. If you sit down and relax for a moment, the prior language will pop out the same as it always did. You must make a special effort to turn the new language into almost a mother tongue, into a habit. Then the change becomes a routine and does not require constant effort. Only from time to time, when you do not pay enough attention, the old language would sprout like remnants of an accent of an old immigrant.

The important part is accepting that your old thinking tools do not necessarily serve you well or that they include a certain bug that prevents you from moving forward.

There are a few difficulties in defining friendly thinking.
How can we make a distinction between reciting from a blocked brain, searching through various drawers in the brain and retrieving information from them, and brain activity which we call thinking and a creation of the brain?

To what extent can we trust that section of the brain we call the landlord, the one which is supposed to channel our brain into friendly thinking? We create this section in our brain and through our brain. So it is somewhat problematic as any body that appoints the body that inspects and supervises it. It seems prejudiced from the start. In general, the organs of the brain and the thinking avoid definitions and even understanding. The numerous studies which are being carried out around the world suffer from a built-in bug. The weighing of the brain, examination of its texture, its scanning in advanced tools, discovery of complex, extensive electro-chemical activity which accompanies mental processes create the illusion that we are on the verge of revealing the secrets of the brain.

Human attempts to understand and not to leave even a single area of the brain unexamined are, of course, very welcome. And indeed, these studies are amazing. The problem lies in the hasty interpretations of the findings of the numerous studies. They provide us with "truths" that make it more difficult to understand the brain. These studies do not provide a shred of evidence regarding the cerebral activity called thinking.

A thorough investigation of materials such as plastic, ivory, wood or metal which the chess pawns are made of will not make us any wiser regarding the strategic game of chess, a thorough investigation of the cardboard or plastic cards will not help us understand the sophisticated game of bridge – it is all about the instruments of the game and not the game itself.

The organs of the brain are only the instruments of thinking and not thinking itself.

Something else that is not easy to understand: friendly thinking does not have to be right. It only must be orientated towards starting a friendly process. For instance, a woman who is stuck and suffering was asked to learn how to ride a motorcycle. Retroactively, it turned out that after she had mastered the ability to ride, she added more and more abilities, and after a short while she made an enormous change in her life and the life of her family. But we must not forget that this is an insight post factum. The other possibility was that she would learn how to ride a motorcycle and then get herself killed in a road accident.

Friendship

A production that includes three components: enjoying others' ability, enabling others to enjoy our ability and a collection of abilities with a whole greater than the sum of its parts.

A molecule of friendship is a situation in which someone expresses his ability and someone else receives it. It is not clear who enjoys it the most the "cow or the calf"; it is also not clear who does a bigger favor, the one who gives or the one who receives and grants the opportunity to express. A person who gives and then feels deprived or exploited misses the sense of satisfaction that derives from the ability to give. A person who wants to give will always find a person who will enjoy it. If you do not find a person who needs your love, you will discover that cute puppies never refuse love.

In a friendly deal two people complete one another in a more symmetric manner. They add to each other and receive from each other mutually as in a barter. Each one gives his friend something he is missing. When the friendly deal broadens and becomes friendship, more and more components are included in it until two people become **experts** of each other. They notice not only the abilities of themselves and the other, but also their weaknesses and limitations. They add to each other without burdening one another. Thus, they play an important part in each other's life.

When your identity includes another person it means an enormous change of identity has taken place. If you wish, this is what love is all about. Learning to love is at the top of all our abilities.

Nevertheless, considering the weaknesses of others is not always friendly. Sometimes, the one who takes advantage of his position within the relationship in order to produce change without considering the weakness of the other does a friendly deed; in such a case, even if the processes of change burden the spouse or the partner at first, he remains persistent, the partner might eventually join the change. I see this type of burdening as a positive one.

Let's take **for example** a woman who loves to dance and who thinks her spouse might enjoy moving himself on the dance floor – but he refuses, that is, he rejects the opportunity she offers him. (What is unfriendly? To stand by him gloomy and complaining, as if he is the reason you are not dancing because it kills the stimulation or to pass the time with a friend because by doing so you become too predictable). The woman goes out without him and chooses to dance with a nice man who is a superb dancer; and when the spouse finds that the woman enjoys dancing even without him it might make him change his mind and join her. (It might also make him angry, but if she is not too concerned, she will declare that a person who tries **to prevent** her from doing what she likes cannot possibly be her friend.)

The burden she imposed on him has led to a friendly production – going dancing together. Obviously the pinnacle of production is a change in entertaining quality. She is not supposed to make do with a situation in which her spouse forces himself and comes dancing with her unenthusiastically. Only at the beginning of the process we will compromise enjoyment. Later on, he is supposed to start enjoying the activity. If he is incapable of enjoying it, he will have to be replaced with a person with a much better ability. This type of burden promotes the welfare of both partners and it is friendly even when the other side does not produce change, since, at least, one of the partners is granted a pleasant opportunity to develop and does not limit himself out of consideration for a declining spouse.

In general it is best to avoid complaining, not to preach or tell adults what to do and what not to do. It is not friendly since, as aforementioned, it kills stimulations and decreases the wish to act. It is especially true when it comes to teenagers who tend to rebel. **Instead of telling an adult what to do, it is preferable to place data**, namely, to tell the other side what **you** are about to do, or just to do what you have decided you should do. It might trigger the other side to move forward, and, in any case, it will make you partner take you into consideration.

In certain cases you place data and take a big chance. Meaning, you make it clear for the other person that he cannot remain the same and remain a friend of yours at the same time. So that if the other person chooses not to change, he loses your friendship. It is a friendly deed for two reasons. First, if you are important to the other person, it will make him produce change. If you are not that important to him, at least you send away a person who imposes a great burden on you. a person who does not take you into consideration .Obviously such a crude means should be used only with the most extreme behaviors. Anyway, the expectations that adults would change should not be too high. However, it is exactly the opposite when it comes to children. Here it is considered a missing if the parents do not do whatever they can in order to produce desirable changes for the sake of their children. I recommend parents to start with a fun period so that the children would have a considerable baggage. Since in unfriendly relationships the child has nothing to lose. On the contrary, if you push him away, he will enjoy it more.

Thus, friendship does not mean to stand aside ant not to react. You should do whatever you can in order to encourage your friend to make a friendly change. The guides in Friendship School do not have any enforcement means to force a student to do what he should do. They can only try to persuade him, and if they do not succeed, they should send the decliner home.

In mature friendship, you prefer the other person's welfare to his love. Pleasing him, in this case, means to prefer yourself, to fulfill your own need to be loved and accepted.

Long friendships are worthy and we should use them in a friendly manner. For instance, an old, good friend of mine had been considered asthmatic for many years and it had been known that physical exercise might lead to a severe attack. I persuaded him to join me for walks and joggings on the beach. He obviously said that he is incapable of doing that, but I did not give in. For the last two decades he has been thin, muscular and totally healthy. He is free of the disease which I doubt he ever had. He is also an example of a student who became better than the teacher. Friendship is a profession that can be studied and acquired. It is an essential capability since it constitutes the basis for success in every aspect of life. I believe it is a "must subject" since we operate inside a human fabric in every area of our lives. Some of us studied this subject in their first school - their parents house, if they were lucky enough to be raised by people who knew how to enjoy each other. The ones who were not that lucky should intentionally add this ability to themselves. A poor ability in the present might turn into an expertise in the future. A person who did not bother to learn this ability will find it difficult to form a relationship with another person. A person who neglected his abilities in this area and stopped nurturing them, is doomed to lose his ability to enjoy himself in the presence of other people. If we wish to befriend another person, we should first refer to our reservoir of abilities and then to the other's reservoir of abilities and ask ourselves what we can add to it. The aim is not do a good deed such as helping an old lady cross the street, but a complex relationship which takes the other person and his abilities into account. In addition, we should ask ourselves how we can enjoy the other's abilities. As far as friendship with children is concerned, we might avoid using our abilities in order to let the child develop his abilities. Taking advantage of each other's possibilities contributes to a strong, rewarding friendship.

We must remember that our resources are limited and thus even when it comes to friendship we should decide who will enjoy more of our time and who will remain within the group of not so close friends. Moreover, different connections amongst people and interests are also an expression of friendly abilities. Identifying possible connections and mixes contributes to the development of a friendly community.

In addition, I would like to point out that in my opinion, friendship does not necessarily means meeting with people. Friendship means the entire process of expansion of our ability and our world. If, for example, we have not learnt to swim and enjoy the water, and perhaps we are even afraid of the water, learning how to swim is, in my opinion, acquiring the ability to befriend the sea and the swimming pool. Investing in yourself and nurturing your abilities constitutes a friendly approach towards yourself, and towards others as well.

The more equipped you are, the more you are able to contribute to other people. In Friendship School we highly recommend to develop the ability of befriending, not only in order to make friends and meet spouses, but also since this ability constitutes the basis of successful partnerships, businesses, and organization of manpower. Personally, I believe that developing this ability from a very young age, also guarantees the survival of human race – since the dangerous rejection means which are common in limited and fundamentalist cultures have the power to destroy life on earth.

Homework

An operating and application system of the processes of change and development which is, in fact, the important part of change production.

The term "homework" is as important as the term "Friendship School" and it is designed to show the student that he is here to learn, and that he is not here for a therapy. We believe that traditional psychological sessions are not efficient. The benefit mainly derives from what the patient does between sessions and that means homework.

I am not trying to be modest. An accompaniment by a guide from Friendship School makes the process shorter. The guide, with his familiarity and understanding, can easily pinpoint repressions and crude rejections of the client and this is certainly useful. Participation in the workshop also contributes a great deal. However, it should be noted that the most important thing is the homework. If a person comes to the meetings but does not do anything in between, he will not benefit and will probably be expelled from school.

Homework is based on our days' content. We shape our days and decide what to plant in them. Things that are not included in our days' content do not exist as far as we are concerned. Thus, if we wish to develop something, we are supposed to devote some time for it on a daily basis; this is our homework. For example, if we wish to develop our relationships, we should meet friends; if we wish to improve our piano playing, we should combine tapping the keys in our schedule. If we do not do the homework, our wishes will remain limited to **our imagination**. A person who convinces himself he does not have time actually says that his timetable was forced upon him. It is not so – we are the masters of our time. Only at a prison dungeon there is not enough maneuvering space to select one's occupations. In order to plan the homework schedule we must think of our reservoir of abilities. On the one hand, we should not burden ourselves with unrealistic tasks, but, on the other hand, we should not deal with things which are too easy for us, and thus, do not add anything to our reservoir of abilities. A person who reaches a conclusion after a single meeting has not even started to do his homework. Every new element we add to our world requires a **set of experiences**, before we do some self search and decide what to keep and what to leave behind. A person who has not built his identity yet, should experience several fields simultaneously. A few weeks later he should make comparisons, prefer and reduce. How do we plan friendly homework? This is a personal question which demands customization. One person should do homework related to delinquency and another should focus on sports. Another person is required to make coffee for his mother and befriend her. Should we start studying Italian? We have to ask ourselves if it is worthwhile for us, or is it better to invest our efforts in something else. We should check how it relates to the other components of our identity; check whether we neglect something else which is more important to us. In other words, perhaps a crude rejection of a more important goal is hidden behind our desire to study Italian and it will remain further neglected.

Anyway, all the things we agree on are supposed to be reflected in the homework. If you are a single man who wants to be in a relationship, it should be reflected in your daily routine through numerous relevant experiences. If your time is filled up with various occupations, but not with the occupation you are supposed to focus on, you are not doing relevant homework.

You wish to become a painter who enjoys his art and makes a living from it; you should paint on a daily basis.

At our school one is not allowed to say: "I wish" without expressing it in practice, through homework. We will not mislead ourselves that we are about to see the north, when we are headed southward, or toward any other direction which is not north.

Identity

A reservoir of all the things we gather through our life time. Another version: The answer to the question "Who am I?" according to our abilities.

There are factors that define our identity against our will. For example, we cannot choose our place of birth. However, once we become mobile we are able to move in all directions and to decide to settle in a different place and to shape a new identity for ourselves. When we grow up we are able to change the name given to us by our parents to a more desirable name. If we wish, we can get rid of numerous characterizations forced upon us and shape our identity according to our choice.

In the course of life sometimes a person comes across circumstances which force him to make changes in his identity. When a person is fired from his job, he is sometimes forced to change his profession. A disaster might force a person to start from scratch. Sometimes a person rehabilitates his own identity, and sometimes he builds himself a new world and a new identity.

Immigration to another country requires enormous changes. Some people try to maintain their old identity. Some combine in their identity characteristics that were not typical of them in their birth country. An Israeli immigrant, for instance, might start going to the synagogue on Saturday. If an immigrant remains the same in the new country, does it mean that he is loyal to his identity or that he is a learning decliner? In my opinion, a Jewish or Israeli or Muslim ghetto reflects disability more than free will. When I observe some of the ultra-orthodox people in Jerusalem who wear clothes that were appropriate in cold countries in east Europe, it seems like learning declining. Selecting what to take from our old identity and what to add to it is a complicated scholastic deed of shaping our identity. People who are used to the scholastic culture, especially small children, absorb almost immediately the language of the new place in addition to their mother tongue. Sometime the new language becomes as dominant as the mother tongue. Sometimes it even becomes more dominant . Thus, a complicated identity which is hard to define is developed. An Israeli who has lived in France for about twenty years becomes, to a large extent, a French. But he will not be French as a French person who has never been an Israeli. If he comes to live in Israel again he will not come home to his old identity. He would find out that the country has changed and that he, at least for a certain period, is an immigrant in his homeland. Even when he speaks Hebrew, his language will be a bit archaic and he will speak in a French accent. Let's make it even more complicated. Suppose your son marries a non-Jewish woman, from Lebanon. Will their children be Jewish, Israeli, Arabs, Catholics???

Thus, it is not easy to define a person's identity according to the nationality, the religion or the ethnic group in a changing social reality.

In spite of all of the above, it must be noted that most people in the world are never exposed to questions of identity. A person who was born in an ultra-orthodox family and studied at ultra-orthodox institutions, inherited an identity when he was born. Surely, it happens that from time to time, especially during adolescence, someone rebels against his destiny, finds a new path and shapes a different identity, but most people belong to their community and do not ask too many questions. Most of them are even proud of themselves as if they have won the best possible identity.

Similarly, most people live all their lives in one place, almost disconnected to the rest of the world. Progress has not reached them, and even if it did, they would refer to it as a disruption to their right way of life.

There is no doubt that upheavals have caused significant changes of identity among people who came across special circumstances. It is also known that sometimes people make changes in their identity. A religious person might become secular. A secular person might become religious and his whole life changes. A single person gets married. Young people become parents. A smoker becomes a non-smoker. A non-smoker becomes a smoker. A homosexual becomes heterosexual or bisexual. A heterosexual leaves his family and becomes a homosexual. A landlord becomes homeless. A healthy person becomes ill or disabled. A living person commits suicide and becomes dead.

All of the above prove that it is possible to change one's identity, for better or worse, depending on the beholder. The ability to shape our identity exists.

Many people define identity according to profession, prominent characteristics, such as appearance or likability, or according to measurements that were determined based on awkward diagnosis. All of these definitions are not accurate.

We recommend a definition that derives from the major occupations of the person. Obviously defining the identity according to capabilities is not completely thorough, but it is better than the other definitions.

As mentioned before, in scholastic culture a person is committed to the ongoing process of shaping his identity. And later on becomes committed to nurturing his identity, and if the need arises, to reinvent himself.

I allow myself to use a somewhat judgmental tone here. In scholastic culture the person develops the core of his identity and more and more branches grow in the process. The branches are additional occupations and part-time hobbies that enrich the main occupations, the ones that take up most of the identity cake. In most cases these people become experts in certain domains and the additional occupations serve as spices that enrich the dish.

Some people move in all directions, constantly discover new branches and create a tree that spreads sideways and lacks a central trunk that grows upwards. The enjoyment derived from their abilities is partial and numerous stimulations distract and confuse them.

In addition, behaviors which harm the identity are to be taken into account compared with actions that suit it. A parking offence, for instance, does not harm the identity, but sexual harassment might destroy the career of a person with a delicate role as if he had decided to commit suicide in terms of his identity.

The process of shaping the identity is made of the same components needed for producing change. When a person with a serious developmental bug comes to see me, I demand that he spends all his free time doing homework. Otherwise, he will probably keep moving in all directions and destroy unknowingly whatever he has managed to achieve. This is the nature of his bug. This approach is interfering, even intrusive, but it promotes change.

It is hard to describe the suffering of a person who has not developed an identity; a person who does not really know himself. At the moment he is a waiter. At the moment he is a student. At the moment he is dating someone, but he does not know who he is and what he will do when he grows up.

Shaping identity takes time. First we should sharpen our basic tools and then we should use them in order to shape our identity. **To locate and identify the better abilities compared to other abilities**, to identify priorities, to promote the things that give us satisfaction and are beneficial to us until our personal identity is shaped.

Many people find it difficult and prefer to establish an immediate identity. To wear army uniforms, police uniforms, a sports team's uniform, religious signs etc. Others establish random identities. They make their living from a temporary job they keep it until they become pensioners. Some marry the first woman they have a relationship with. Perhaps you would claim that they chose not to be exposed to the enormous number of confusing possibilities and to select their identity characteristics.

The life of a person who has an identity is much easier. The identity is the ultimate <u>maximal reduction.</u> Choosing your personal identity from the colorful, endless selection. Choosing your occupation, your companion, the place where you live your life. Knowing what contributes to your identity and what harms it. This kind of person knows what to anticipate when he wakes up in the morning and when he comes home at night. He finds his occupations worthy and he has an automatic screening tool. When such a person knows he is a layer, as he knows his own name, he does not look at doctors or engineers want ads. He does not need to ask himself questions about his identity every morning. He does not need to ask himself what to do and what not to do. Identity contains an automatic mechanism that rejects certain questions in advance and points at other issues. It may seem like repression but it is not. Here, the automatic mechanisms in the brain are not responsible for the screening. The person himself, the shaper of the identity, is the one responsible for it. This is friendly since your strengths are available to be invested in whatever else you choose to invest in. This is one of the origins of the drive to study further which is the main characteristic of people of scholastic culture. It is not crude rejection. People are exposed to the surrounding and sometimes to additional stimulations but these do not lead to identity confusion. Nevertheless, in order not to become immersed in repression, and since the common tendency is to keep the routine, even if it is a good routine, it is important to raise identity questions from time to time and to perform a kind of soul search in order to make sure our identity has not become a trap of blocking automatic repression. Do not hesitate to perform occasional soul search. The existing foundation makes sure we would not be confused by every gust of wind. We are knowledgeable about certain domains and thus we will not replace them with inappropriate ones for no reason. On the other hand, we will not miss a special opportunity for change if we are exposed to one which is worthy and can compete with the contents of our old foundation.

A nurtured identity raises the starting point of other stimulations. For example, if someone who has built his professional identity, senses a stimulation to add another occupation in his free time, it will be a hobby related to his profession. If he chooses the new interest over the old one, it should probably be worth it.

A friendly attitude towards our identity requires not only wide and comprehensive contextual understanding, but also identifying growth processes and possible scenarios. Repression of the expected future is not less damaging than repression of current abilities. For instance, if someone has built her identity based merely on being a pretty girl, she will find out in the future that age bites into such an identity mercilessly. In other words, her identity has no future. Prettier young women will push her aside. Another example is an excellent athlete who finds out at a pretty young age that he is too old for this competitive sport. In other words, people who do not develop a more complex identity with a potential to grow, will soon lose their purpose of life or suffer endlessly due to the things they cannot achieve. On the other hand, a person who has prepared an infrastructure for possible growth will build the layers of his identity till his last day. The athlete will become a coach, a business man, a movie star, a director or choose any other occupation which is not limited to very young people. The pretty girl will became a layer, a writer, a counselor and the list is endless.

Immediate Relief

An immediate response to stimulation.
In general, the immediate relief is an automatic reaction which is crude and nondiscriminatory. The relief provides quick easement; thus, the means through which we achieve quick, liberating relief are tempting and addicting: tears, sorrow, shouts, as well as drugs, alcohol, medications, and food, watching TV, computer games and the like.

People who have poor learning abilities and cannot express themselves sufficiently have a greater tendency to become addicted to various pastimes which do not require any efforts. People who know how to learn and develop more sophisticated abilities get pleasure and satisfaction from self-expression. Genuine satisfaction, after all, contains an abundance of relief.

Contrary to the common opinion, I believe that **it is much easier to suffer than to enjoy life**. Any fool knows how to find relief in insults, fights and shouts; you do not need to learn it. However, developing the ability to enjoy, requires special investment. It is much more difficult to learn how to enjoy playing the piano than finding a liberating relief in crying and anger, insult and jealousy. We are all familiar with the daily dilemma: should we watch TV or practice our musical instrument? Should we play a computer game or study for a test? The struggle is between investment and efforts which will be beneficial in the long run and an immediate, quick reward. At the crossroads of opportunities, we have to choose between channels that provide addictive, immediate relief and prevent us from growing, and channels that require effort that will achieve a superb ability and enable self-expression. When a person's energy leaks through the faucets of relief, he usually lacks the energy to invest in learning which will enable more rewarding achievements. I find most means of immediate relief negative, especially when they are addictive and thus damage the identity of the user. Let's take for example a talented actor who is also a drinker and tends to get into quarrels. Such an actor is considered unreliable, and directors will be reluctant to hire him for important productions. And if it is a person who does not have a professional identity, he will be defined by his means of relief – drug addict, drunk, violent etc.

A person who is already addicted to means of negative relief, even if decides to change all of the sudden, will find it difficult. Until he manages to create tools for enjoying himself and his occupations – a process that takes time – he will be forced to find relief through his regular, immediate means.

On the other hand, I certainly do not recommend rehabilitation acts and restraint. The popular rehabilitation methods take up much energy and only a few are able to be persistent and to succeed. We should also consider the danger that the restraint will eventually lead to an uncontrolled outbreak. In Friendship School I recommend joining **all** forces to creating new abilities. Promoting abilities in areas which enable us to express ourselves enjoyably constitutes an efficient solution whose entertaining quality competes well with that of the addictive activity. Addiction to bridge, for example, easily defeats other addictions such as addiction to TV or gambling.

In order to increase the success rate of the process, one should use many **positive immediate relief means** which are taken from the personal reservoir of abilities: walks, jogging, any type of gymnastics, dancing, singing, sexual activity and the like. Such activities provide the body and soul with a gratifying immediate relief which is sufficient for a couple of hours, without causing damage to the identity and make it easier for us to promote the selected expression channel.

Sometimes a person becomes addicted to a positive immediate relief such as sports and neglects his prior plans of becoming a doctor or a pianist. I still believe that an addiction to sports is much more preferable than a negative addiction.

A person who learns to derive enjoyment from the things he does, can easily share other people's happiness. He is able to enjoy their ability even if it is better than his. Accepting the other's ability contributes a lot to the production of friendship, companionship and love. On the other hand, a person who is negatively triggered, tends to make comparisons, suffers from comparing himself to others, becomes disappointed and imposes a burden on others.

Junction of Opportunities

An encounter between our current state and the things we are exposed to. The point from which we scan the scenery in front of us and learn to select our desirable targets and the course which will take us there safely.

The junction of opportunities does not necessarily have to be a crossroads in which we cannot choose between studying medicine or law, between getting married and remaining single or between staying in our country or relocating to another country. Our daily life is full of junctions of opportunities. For instance, to identify the relevant stimulus, to choose among numerous stimulations we are exposed to the one stimulation we want to focus on. Should we be tempted by a certain immediate relief or should we choose another direction which promotes us? At the junction we sometimes choose the computer game or a lazy wandering with friends, and sometimes we muster enough energy to do our homework or prepare for a test.

We made the choice. In a little while we will find ourselves in front of a new junction of opportunities where we will have to make another choice. The most difficult junction, the almost **fatal** one is at the **beginning** of the process of producing change. Here we must do activities which are totally opposite from the way we feel or think. For instance, we have decided to lose some weight, to add sports activities to our daily routine and to walk a few kilometers in the mornings before going to work. We enrolled in the gym. We have done these activities once or twice and were very pleased with ourselves. And then, all of the sudden, we feel we cannot go on. Terrible fatigue, various scary pains, we must undergo some medical tests. Perhaps we are unable to wake up in the morning. If we are tempted to stay in bed, we will repeat the school year; remain at the same place, unchanged.

How can we find the strength to stand up?

We have made an appointment and as time goes by, the excitement and expectation turn into weariness and reluctance. Again, we find ourselves at a critical junction – where should we turn? Which side to choose? Should we choose our side or the side of the symptoms of crude rejection and various side effects?

We have covered some distance but we cannot celebrate change yet. Another wave of different symptoms arrives accompanied by doubts. You have been living together for a month and the things you found interesting become boring and oppressive. What happened? You want to let go. You have bought workout equipment and after a while it turns into a clothes hanger. You have almost finished writing your partnership contract and at the last minute you get cold feet and cancel it.

You have been studying for four years and are about to get your degree. All of the sudden you feel you do not like what you are doing and want to quit.

I do not claim that you must finish whatever you have started, but when we scan the scenery, there is a difference between a scenario in which you find out the studies do not suit you at the beginning of the process and turn to another direction and a scenario in which you almost reach the end of the course and are about to enjoy the fruit of your hard work.

This is the reason that in Friendship School we search for every possible, sophisticated device that can assist us with a friendly production. Management, getting help from a capable person etc. It is very difficult to ensure a journey free of mistakes. Here and there you might **lose a battle** or two, but you must make sure you eventually win the **war**. You have made a change in your identity and it cannot be taken away from you. You will not be discouraged by any gust of wind. You have moved to the next stage.

See: "Opportunity."

Language of Communication

All the verbal and behavioral thinking and expression tools at our disposal through which we express ourselves.

This language of communication is also the manner in which we perceive reality, decode it, and grant meaning to it. There are many different types of communication languages.

Mother Tongue: Our first language of communication is totally accidental. Nobody chooses his biological parents or the place in which he is born. Thus the English learn English, and the Chinese learn Chinese whether they like it or not.

The Language of Culture: The set of values and symbols which is at the basis of our behavior. We learn to pronounce sounds the same way we learn to love, hate, sense, think and evaluate in accordance with the culture we live in. From the period of childhood on, we learn to like a certain pop-star and to hate oriental music, to believe in the Torah and to hate Arabs, to judge what is pretty and what is ugly, etc.

In most cases, during normal developmental process we are exposed to additional cultural opportunities and acquire a remarkable ability which enables us to see things from different point of views. People who have developed learning abilities are capable of understanding and accepting people who are different from them alongside people who resemble them. A person who activates his learning ability and learns other languages of culture besides the one he is used to, creates an opportunity for negotiation and a possibility for encounters and change. Such a person does not find it hard to live with people who speak a different language of culture – Arabs, religious people, seculars, Buddhists and so forth. A person who remains with a single language of culture is like a person who stays in kindergarten for decades, refuses to develop and is not even curious to know what other people have. He is like a fish in an aquarium and every change in the water temperature or type of food jeopardizes its existence. He can only live in a single environment and does not enjoy the magnificent human capability of changing and expanding one's world by studying various languages of communication. **Learning means adding something new to yourself**; something you have not liked or known previously. Such an addition expands the identity. A person who is limited to a single language of communication is able to communicate only with people who speak that language. This is the reason why singles usually feel good in the company of other singles, homosexuals seek the company of other homosexuals who think and behave like them and religious people prefer praying at a synagogue where everybody knows the same version of prayers. It is not difficult to make a distinction between an act of thinking and discretion of a person who is willing to learn various languages of communications and a predictable recitation of a person who uses only his familiar language of communication and in spite of the ever-changing reality, his opinion on the reality never changes.

The Language of Love, The Language of Friendship: The manners in which we express love or friendship to the other and the manners in which the other expresses his love or friendship to us.

There are many different languages of love. When we build a relationship with a spouse it is important to know the manners in which the other expresses his love to us and to show the other our expression means. Many mishaps at the beginning of relationships derive from misunderstandings caused by the fact that every person judges the other according to his personal language of love and every person is ignorant when it comes to the many other languages of love. It is true also for the language of friendship; if we wish to create a bond with a different person – we should better learn this person. If we do not know how to study, and the other must always adjust to us, it greatly reduces the chances of creating a successful relationship.

It is such a shame to make do with our first language of love and be limited to it. In a normal process of growth, people expand their ability to love and be loved. Even if a person is born into a culture in which hugs and caresses are exceptional, he can easily add the missing ability to himself whether by taking private lessons from a friend who likes to hug or by joining a workshop of experimenting touch after which he would be able to hug and caress and be hugged and caressed.

The Language of Complaints: An agreed language between two people who agree not to enjoy each other, to seek each others' weaknesses, to defend and attack. This is the formal language in the land of guilt and it is extremely widespread. The speakers of this language outnumber the speakers of the Chinese language.

The speakers of this language are convinced they are interested in making a change in their lives, and that if only people listen to their justified complaints, everything will be better. The truth is that they are learning decliners, stuck in one place. They communicate with the environment only in this language. Unfortunately, they have an audience that listens to them and identifies with them. In the audience one may find psychologists who make their living from listening and contribute to a ritual in which every nonsense ostensibly turns into a fact. Thus, the complaints are recorded and perpetuated in the participants' consciousness.

In practice, the language of complaints is one of the most lethal rejection means. The owner of the complaint always hits something. **He abolishes the existing elements through the non-existing ones**. Indeed, similar to other languages, as long as two people communicate in the same language, no change is to be expected. The first person who starts speaking in a different language gives change a chance.

The Language of Facts: A language which is based on actions and not on talks, emotions or impressions. In fact, any person, in any encounter on earth, cannot avoid a situation in which his brain is filled with impressions and diagnosis regarding himself and the people around him. However, we must all avoid making a diagnosis or be able to get rid of an impression which was fixated in our brain a long time ago. It is important that we let the facts, and not the words or emotions, speak for themselves. We should see what the person in front of us **does** and only based on a **prolonged** observation, make our own diagnosis. Too often there is a significant gap between the things a person tells about himself and the things he does. Sometimes his words are characterized by underestimation and depression while in fact he has managed to do some quite impressive things in his life. Sometime a person speaks of himself as if he were a tiger, while his abilities are extremely limited. Thus, an observation of the things a person does constitutes a more reliable source of friendly negotiations. At our school written homework is very common and so are the day's content, meeting reports etc.

Using the language of facts teaches us to refer to ourselves in a truthful manner. If we perceive ourselves as liberal parents, for instance, it is time we examine the facts: do we really let our children to do things which do not match our point of view, such as dyeing their hair green?

Leakage

Another way of referring to our mental budget and to where we channel it.
More than once it seems to me that a person claims that he wishes to achieve something which seems achievable to me, but instead of trying to achieve it, the person leaks to all directions till he is unable to achieve his proclaimed goal. It is based on the image of water flowing through the pipe, leaking from different holes and all is left is a weak flow from the tap.
See: "Relevant Stimulus," "Passing Time" and "Management."

Learning Decliner

A person who uses all his might, usually unconsciously, to prevent learning and change.
When people ask me during lectures what the success rate of my method is I usually say – close to a hundred percent. But it is so because I select my clients. Learning decliners do not have a place at our school. These people use all their might to prevent learning and change; and we, the guides or therapists, do not have enforcement means to force another person to invest in change. As we all know, there is no law against stupidity. On the contrary, sometimes it seems that stupidity has a high rating. In addition there are no laws that force a person to be happy. On the contrary, many people are used to being unhappy. Most of the **supportive** systems that support people who have problems mostly support themselves. It could be

claimed that numerous people make their living from people who create problems and suffer from them.

A learning decliner is someone who has to repeat the school year, sometimes for decades. He feels the same as if time went by him. And if he does undergo change, it is not initiated by him, but due to a traumatic event.

In Friendship School we associate with people who choose to nurture their abilities rather than their problems. If we come across learning decliners, we look for people who can influence them to produce change, and only if it is not possible, we give up and send the learning decliners home.

Parents of small children have enormous power that enables them to produce changes in their children. Close spouses are also powerful enough to promote change.

See: "Friendship."

Learning Workshops

Effective meetings in which the participants share their abilities and urge one another to succeed.

These workshops are not similar to the various "support groups" that have become very popular lately and that consist of people who share the same problem such as compulsive eaters, ex-alcoholics, victims of anxiety. I see these workshops as a cultural ghetto. Surely the sharing creates a convenient, acceptive atmosphere for those who participate in the workshops but it also allows them not to change. The fact that they publicly share experiences of anxiety, or the hardships of diet and support each other makes them trample together in the same swamp. Sometimes the group even worsens their situation; while participants report about their difficulties, distresses and deterioration, they might drag the others along with them. This is true also for support group which do not necessarily deal with a common problem. Single mothers, for example, will find themselves focusing on obstacles and not on success. If someone happens to change to the extent that he no longer needs the group, he could be considered a traitor.

In the **learning** workshops, on the other hand, the common denominator of the participants is not a difficulty, but ability. When capable people meet other capable people, who are sometimes even more capable than them, they are stimulated to improve their ability as well. They are asked to share their progress and not their problems with the others. The group pressure urges the members of the group to move forward. In such a workshop there are plenty of means to develop managements with the others. There are plenty of production accessories. Common transactions simplify the various productions as opposed to a situation when a person is supposed to make the effort all by himself. Such a workshop urges change. A person who is stuck gets help from another member who is able to show him how to move forward. Later on, he will guide others.

Low Self Image

The popular tendency to undermine ourselves which have been serving for many years as an excellent source of income for the canonical therapists.

See: "Dealing with Problems."

Management

A tool which enables us to organized our time in the best way.

Deciding which activities will be included in our schedule and the ways in which this decision is implemented is what I call "management." Obviously when we plan our schedule, we must consider constraints which cannot be ignored. But, with the help of correct management, we will not miss the opportunity to make the best of our lives. Most of our time will be dedicated to things we like and choose, and minimal time will be dedicated to constraints. What else can we do with constraints? We might even learn to like some of the constraints which will better their entertaining quality. For instance, it is possible to turn house cleaning into something which is not that horrible by playing pleasant music and getting help from a few friends. Another option is to offer our services in something we like to do and using the money for hiring a housemaid. Another friendly way is to compensate an unpleasant constraint by planning a special pastime. For instance, if we must undergo an unpleasant dental treatment, we can plan special pastimes before and after the treatment. Thus, we will have a nice day in spite of the constraint. A vacation with a friend, for those are not accustomed to that, will be much more successful with the help of planning. It is a well known medication for eliminating arguments.

Again, we will emphasize that the ones who are used to obligations and constraints and are perceived as the ones who carry the burden, are capable of making a significant identity change more easily than others. They should use their magnificent ability to carry the burden for the sake of completely different cultural elements. **It means using an existing ability for the sake of acquiring a new one**. For example, an individual who has great working abilities and can work long hours in a row quite easily, can use this ability at home as well. In other words, in the past he used to come home exhausted and too mentally drained for his wife and children, now he comes home as if he has not finished his work day. It is like making a switch which keeps him committed for a short while after he has entered the door. A person that does this homework for a while finds out, soon enough, that he can enjoy himself with the wife and the children as well. Similarly, people who are not used to enjoying a vacation should refer to their first vacations as an essential work. If they are patient enough, they will soon find out that their abilities broaden and enable them both to work and to enjoy vacations.

Management is an arbitrary act. It is based on a decision rather than on desires. And why does it contribute to producing change? Since many beginnings involve an effort which is not that enjoyable. For instance, practicing a complicated shift from one accord to the other when playing a certain musical instrument. And sometimes dozens or hundreds of irritating rehearsals are needed before the music flows. Not many will be persistent enough to go through the difficult and not so interesting part and they, in fact, would give up the reward – which is the ability to play and produce music, which is one of the most marvelous pleasures a person might have. Similarly, a person who wants to play tennis is required to practice countless forehand and backhand strokes in order to achieve the pure pleasure felt by those who already know how to play tennis.

Management requires a set of **productions** from theory to practice. It is also an important layer of sharpening tools for identity formation. First we should practice management for the next couple of days: what can be done tomorrow afternoon, and what can and should be done tomorrow evening. The more complicated identity issues should be faced later: what should be my profession, and what should be my hobby, whom to marry, whom to befriend etc.

The resolved objectors of management are the "spontaneous". They want to do whatever they feel like whenever they feel like it and do not agree to plan meetings and pastime in advance. Out of shortsightedness they perceive themselves as free as long as they do not commit. In most cases these people are contended with little. They act according to various moods and accidental caprices. They get bored easily and must be in constant move, mostly sideways and not forward. It is difficult for them to reach rich experiences that are reached by persistence and delving into a particular field. Their friends see them as unreliable. A dual or multiple production requires many efforts and fails most of the time. For instance, finding several people who are hungry at the same time and available for a meal, or several people who would want to go dancing spontaneously without prior arrangements.

A person who is used to management will find out that even without it and in a spontaneous manner, he is able to produce a lovely weekend for his family and himself without prior planning. He enjoys the fruits of his persistence and has many options to choose from easily and rapidly. In front of him there are many clear paths in which he has walked before. And he does not need to use a map in an area he has toured numerous times before.

Here and there there are spontaneous people who succeed even without prior planning. But usually they are very famous or very rich. These kind of people easily find people who adjust to their caprices and do as they please. And they enjoy the illusion of satisfaction and success.

But, in most cases, reliable people prefer to befriend other reliable people and make plans with them.

The ones who have abilities will not respond positively to unreliable people. They know that planning in advance enables them to be more sufficient.

See "Production."

Maximal Reduction

A key concept in the shaping of our identity. Reduction of our field of consciousness to the appropriate size which will enable maximal conditions for self-expression when we already have an ability to express ourselves, or convenient conditions for learning the ability when we do not have it.

The term maximal reduction sounds paradoxical since the word "reduction" is usually perceived as negative, but in the frame of the friendly approach it does not have any valued significance. As we cannot possibly be in different places at the same time, we cannot possibly refer to all the stimulations all at once. We must sort them out and find the best reduction which enables us to achieve convenient conditions for learning or to reach sufficient expression.

For instance, when we lack sexual experience it is difficult for us to be aware of the sensations at the tips of our fingers when we caress our partner and of the touch of our partner's hands on our body at the same time. At first, it is best to reduce the elements in order to be able to focus on the sensation, to enjoy it thoroughly and only then to expand the circle of stimulations. We should start touching each other in the dark, in order to focus solely on the sensation of touch; then we should add more and more experiences. Sexual experience, like any other experience, should be built gradually and in a friendly atmosphere. It is not healthy to try to lift a ton; it is better to divide the ton into smaller units and carry them one by one.

The principle of a successful production of change is going step by step. You better first produce a change in your relationship with a young child, and only then try to produce change in the relationship with an adult. If you feel that the responsibility of being a parent is too much for you, you should first practice on a little pet.

From time to time you come to consult with us about choosing your professional identity. We start with slowly, and only later we deal with the heavy, more complicated questions of identity.

Every so often someone who is extremely eager to produce an essential change in his life arrives. Unfortunately there is no escape from preparing a better foundation for the production of change. For a while we would practice on focusing on attentive listening to music or reading a book until we manage to enjoy it and love it. Then we can expose ourselves to loving another person.

Yet, the process of learning is not always linear: sometimes it is better to start with an especially difficult challenge which will pave the way to many easier changes.

It is not that simple to know the level of reduction that suits us. A person who reduces his world too much, will see only part of the scenery and miss the spectrum of opportunities. A person who goes for too many elements will also miss the opportunity of becoming an expert in a field which is suitable for him. Thus, it is a dynamic concept and we must conduct a thorough examination time and time again in order to ensure our maximal reduction is indeed maximal – not too small and not too big.

The discretion involved in finding our maximal reduction is a constant question of identity: where should we invest most of our energies, and what are the things we should give up; what will become our main occupation, what will become a complimentary hobby and what should we give in altogether.

We must examine it with every person according to his personal state of aggregation and learning ability.

Mental Budget

The amount of energy and capabilities at our disposal at every given time.

Mental budget, like physical shape or financial budget is subject to change. A person who has limited mental budget is capable of little. It does not allow him "both." For example, it is hard for him both to study and to work. Obviously, he cannot love a woman, raise children, work, study and find time for a few hobbies.

A devoted scholar increases the abilities and mental budget at his disposal. Thus he has a greater mental budget and as busy as he is he finds time for more.

Awareness of our abilities includes knowing the mental budget at our disposal at every given moment. When someone does not notice he has reached the end of his ability and remains, for instance, in the company of his wife and children, he will eventually be forced to react with crude means such as by yelling or arguing in order to escape from them. Later on, he will have to spend his resources trying to make peace with them. Another person, who is more attentive to his mental budget, will spend an hour with them and then move on to a different occupation, while maintaining a friendly atmosphere. When he recovers, he will meet them again. Obviously, in the context of friendly thinking we aspire to increase our abilities and our mental budget. We will also develop a socio-economic comprehension, which enables economic use of the mental budget. Let's take for example a woman who meets a guy in the South, with whom she likes to travel. She meets another guy in the North with whom she prefers to have sexual intercourse. She also meets a friend in Jerusalem with whom she likes to talk. This woman spends a lot of time on the road. Her energies are directed to different places and she does not improve her ability to make friends. She should find one guy with whom she likes to have sexual intercourse, travel and talk. Then she will be left with enough mental ability to add other friendly components to her life. Other examples of **connecting friendly elements**: finding mutual hobbies together with your spouse, children and friends; going on a long trip with a friend or a spouse - that way you get to see the world and enrich your relationship at the same time

Opportunity

Any event, object or person that comes across our path.
The multiple stimulations we are exposed to constitute the scope of opportunities or field of opportunities. Friendly thinking enables us to seize the opportunity hidden everywhere. If we are part of the scholastic culture and we come across a person who is gathering honey, we will become curious and learn a few things from him.

Namely, the initial reaction towards almost any new thing we are exposed to will be responsiveness, curiosity, interest, stimulation. However, people who are not part of the scholastic culture might react with crude rejection and declare that they are not interested in honey.

Under regular circumstances we are faced with much more opportunities than we can seize and enjoy. For instance, the number of women is enormous, and we cannot possibly refer to them all; there are many more books than we can possibly read; there are many more sites around the world than we can possibly visit. Thus, in Friendship School we dedicate considerable time to sharpening our selection tools. We should learn how to identify the scope of opportunities and to select a handful of things that suit our capabilities. Each one of us is supposed to reach a point I refer to as "blessed troubles," meaning an option to choose between good and good, **or between good and better** and not between good and bad.

In scholastic culture, if we use the example of the honey again, if we remain ignorant of this subject, it is not because we are not interested in the subject, but because we chose to prefer other subjects. With such high-quality tools we could also face events which are perceived as negative and maybe even disastrous. If a certain terrible loss occurs, we will not mourn and agonize, we might even discover that an opportunity arose for something else, perhaps even for a better thing. We will know how to fill the void within us through one of the numerous opportunities surrounding us. If, for example, a person is fired, he might be able to channel himself towards a new job, or towards more interesting occupations.

Production

Designing our weekly schedule, our identity, our life.
I did not choose this term by accident. I would recommend everybody to prepare for producing changes in his life in the same way events

such as movies, series, festivals, parties, birthday parties are produced. A huge force works hard and takes care of dozens, hundreds and even thousands of factors which are supposed to become perfectly united in order to achieve the best end- product.

A production is a link in the chain of <u>management</u>. It is the component that realizes friendly ideas. Achievement of goals requires a long chain of practical productions while moving forward and learning lessons. It includes scanning the cultural, entertaining scenery: performances, lectures, activities and so forth. Long and tiring walks in pursuit of the right place and the right activity. When producing superb <u>entertaining quality</u> with a spouse, the production takes him/her into account when planning the contents of the meetings. For instance, a production is required from a woman who has had only partial relationships, sometimes with multiple partners simultaneously. As part of the production she should go to a party with one of her partners and behave as if they were a married couple. Meaning that they are committed to each other to be at their best. In order for the production to be efficient, it is important to avoid disruption of pre-arranged plans as much as possible. Only two factors can change our production plan: a major failure which is beyond our control or exposure to a worthier opportunity. It is important that our productions succeed and that we do not let any gust of wind (or mood) change our plans.

A production includes the unfolding of several possible scenarios and preparing for each one of them before taking an important step. For example, an important conversation with your teenage daughter requires special consideration. Plan some short phrases that do not include preaching. Try to guess her reaction. Prepare a draft and read it several times. Pick the time and the place which increases the chances of a successful negotiation. For instance, if there is a chance of a conflict, perhaps it is advisable to have the meeting at a coffee-house in a civilized atmosphere instead of meeting at home.

Planning a weekend or an evening for each one of you or for you as a couple is also a common production. The logistics will gradually become an inseparable part of your identity.

As time goes by lessons are learnt and the procedure is upgraded. For instance, if you arrive at the cinema and realize that the tickets are all sold out, or if you arrive at the restaurant and realize that there are no available seats, it is no big deal. The most important thing is that you learn your lesson. Next time, you will buy the tickets and book the seats in advance and your evening will be much more successful. However, when people do not learn the lesson, they make the same mistakes over and over again.

Well, this is quite simple logistics. (It is complicated only to the spontaneous among us and to learning decliners). It is much more complicated to realize decisions such as losing weight. Here, a chain of productions which would eventually lead to an outcome is needed. Changing eating habits and daily diversified sports activities are required. People who are not used to it find it difficult to realize such a decision and many of them fail time and time again. In cases like these sometimes we need to recruit all our means which will enable us to achieve the friendly goal. From associating with different partners to hiring a personal coach. Sometimes we need even more sophisticated and creative means in order to proceed.

See "Homework" and "Day's Contents."

This is a highly important practice which is part of shaping our identity. Only when we are able to persist in numerous productions, in several domains, we are able to compare and identify our priorities, our better capabilities and the relevant opportunities within the field of opportunities. We should not leave the shaping of our identity in the hands of mere chance.

Public Opinion

The reaction of the society surrounding us to our every deed or action.

When we undergo change, we break off the surrounding balance and we can expect various reactions from the people around us. Public opinion has considerable weight which has to be taken into account. One must act with determination in order to overcome the expected resistance. On the other hand, it is also possible to recruit the public opinion to promote desirable things.

Small children identify themselves through grownup's reactions. They will adjust to the public surrounding them. An adult will pave his way along the public opinion, and if necessary, against it.

In most cases the influence of public opinion is negative. It is difficult to be a good pupil in a class in which the popular children are bad pupils. It is not easy to be persistent, to invest efforts and do <u>homework</u> in an environment in which it is customary not to make any efforts. Under the influence of the herd an individual might get trampled and pushed away or be dragged into trampled culture or the culture of diagnosis and judgment. Herding participation in elections and the inflamming of nationalistic emotions are negative results of public opinion. The impact of ratings on the shaping of cultural taste is well known. In such a case a student of the Friendship School is supposed to be able to fight off public opinion in the process of building his identity.

Nevertheless, **it is possible to recruit public opinion to promote abilities.** When we are near people who are important to us, we try to be our best. We are stricter around them than when we are alone. And thus we make the most out of ourselves.

It is clear that we must choose the appropriate social circles. If you choose your single friends and tell them why your last relationship has ended they will encourage you to stay single, not unlike the famous "Seinfeld" team that serves as a support group for chronic singles. Thus, a person that wants to change his identity from a single person to a spouse should expose himself to people who enjoy their family life.

More than once I have mentioned that I help people who have problems only if they are determined to make a change. These people probably have a source which is influenced by past events and produces negative relief. They also have layers of a more developed and determined identity and they make efforts to produce change. On the other hand, when I come across a learning decliner, I will look for a capable person who will serve as audience. Perhaps he will be able to start the process of change.

Sometimes it is the spouse, sometime the parents will be the ones to produce change and sometimes the children will make their parents change. Often bosses and University lecturers are capable of starting the process. To some extent, a friendly end justifies the means.

As far as public opinion is concerned, it is important to know where the borderline is – when the public opinion is a means to producing ability, and when it only limits our identity and suffocates us. The question we should ask is up to what point does the social setting enlarge our identity and enrich us and from what point does it limit and suffocate us? When does our identity as a spouse broaden our identity and when does it limit us? When does the familial setting contribute to the growth of the adolescent and when is he better off without his original family in order to expand his horizons and promote growth?

Sometimes I use the term "audience" to describe the partner to the **language of communication**. The anxious mother, for example, may serve as wonderful audience to the child who causes worry and thus encourages him to take risks. If that is the case, the audience is a negative factor. In other cases the audience is a friendly, enriching factor, for instance, a wife or a mother who likes music may serve as audience that encourages her family members to play music.

Quarrels

A common crude rejection method that is used by spouses who need a rest from each other.
See: "Dealing with Problems."

Relevant Stimulus

The stimulus to which we choose to respond after it has been selected from the countless stimuli surrounding us.
In fact, relevant stimulus is a kind of free choice and it constitutes an important component in the development of our learning ability. Many people give up their independent discretion when they respond to stimuli in an automatic, predictable manner. For instance, when acting according to a certain code of laws or stick to a fixed timetable. Others mix all stimuli and miss them all. It should be noted that at this moment we do not wish to find the answer for complex identity issues and we are not making a soul search or philosophizing about life. At this point we are only interested in practical navigation through the numerous stimuli surrounding us. The relevant stimulus serves as the exact focus within our consciousness. For instance, when you drive a car, the driving and road orientation is the relevant stimulus. All other stimuli are irrelevant. When you are at work, whatever you are supposed to do at work is relevant. All other things are irrelevant. If you are in the middle of a date and are unable to concentrate on your partner, because your mind drifts to another woman, this is not contemplation as is sometime mistakably thought. This is a crude rejection of your date. You destroy whatever you are having at that moment. But when you are alone, thinking of the women, this is contemplation. But here, as well, many people mix things and thus

spend time bothering themselves and not really contemplating. **Contemplation** means scanning two sets of stimuli when each one of them has advantages and disadvantages, and checking which set is better. In reality there are not two identical sets. This is how we learn to choose.

Now I am writing. It means that writing is the relevant stimulus. But I am surrounded by many other stimuli whose aim is to distract me. People, books, TV and of course, countless thoughts running around in different directions. The moment I realize my consciousness has shifted from whatever is relevant, to anything else, I will return it to the appropriate place. This is a basic concentration exercise. Everybody knows it. But if, eventually, I stand up and focus on another stimulus from the ones surrounding me, for instance, I pick up a novel, this novel becomes the relevant stimulus. If I keep reminding myself that I need to write, it will only interrupt with my reading and will not advance my writing. Thus, it is possible to practice and improve our concentration ability and to sharpen our reference tools in the face of irrelevant stimuli.

It is even possible to use constraints which were not chosen and to turn them into relevant stimuli; a mandatory lecture, a role in the army, house cleaning or baby sitting. Friendly discretion tells you that if you are already here you might as well do your homework. To **concentrate** and produce a better entertaining quality. It is better than constantly wishing you were elsewhere. So, you can practice almost anywhere anytime. Some people do arbitrary concentration exercises through meditation; for example, by concentrating on breathing. Obviously there is no harm in that, but I prefer to use whatever exists in our scenery for concentration practice. To tighten our abdominal muscles, to read, to listen to music etc. See <u>Concentration</u>. Our concentration ability precedes our initial contextual awareness. It also precedes the identification of priorities in your identity and life. If he cannot concentrate, he cannot possibly refer to the things that are important to him. Remember that only the ones with the abilities can choose.

Later on, we can use the first rate concentration ability we have acquired and move on to more complex questions. Namely to ask; What the relevant stimulus is or what the friendly stimulus is? What to do first – to organize drawers on Saturday or to spend time with the husband, to read the newspaper or to talk with the child? What to do first and what to do later? The answers to these questions are not given in advance. We will need plenty of practice in order to acquire the ability to make friendly screening and choose the relevant stimulus. In order to do that we must scan the scenery of our options and pinpoint, time and time again, the appropriate stimulus for our maximal ability and the stimulus that promotes whatever is most worthy of promoting at a certain time.

Repression

An act of distraction from one thing to another; often from important fundamental matters to irrelevant things.

This is a basic term in psychology, but I use it differently. Most psychologists use the term "repression" when referring to that mental activity which is meant to remove threatening, unpleasant experiences from the consciousness, and to store them, together with everything else that we wish to forget, in a sort of sealed storage in the brain which is called the sub-consciousness. The psychoanalytic stream and psycho-dynamic approaches which followed it are interested in finding ways of overcoming repression and remembering things that happened in the distant past, based on the assumption that it would release the personality and the strengths within it from heavy burdens and would support change.

These psychologists also refer to the sub-consciousness as the source of interpretation and the basis for insights. If you are late to a meeting with your psychologist, he will tell you that you subconsciously rejecting his dedicated treatment. If you are killed in a road accident, the psychologist will tell your relatives that you probably had a subconscious death wish. I believe that by doing so these psychologists draw the target after the arrow was shot and attribute a meaning to the course of the arrow that did not exist in the first place.

I refer to repression as a **reflex**, which is distraction from important fundamental matters to irrelevant things. When a driver is distracted and pays attention to his friends at the back seat instead of to the road, it is a distraction that might not cause damage on an open, car-free road; and in other cases, on a curved road with a deep abyss, it might lead to a lethal accident. It does not mean that the driver had a hidden death wish. This is merely road distraction.

Similarly, a woman who chooses to fight with her husband and insult him when her little children are present might tell herself she loves her children very much and at the same time that her husband really irritates her. I believe that if she had seen her children, paid attention to their presence, or really loved them, she would not have been able to insult their father in their presence. In this case, repressing the presence of the children causes certain damage and an experience which includes the children would have caused her to postpone the fight with her husband. Following many years of clinical therapy sessions based on the psycho-dynamic approach, I have reached the conclusion that the therapeutic attempt to recall the past – to describe, explain and interpret it – does not contribute to change and even prevent it. In most cases, this pastime comes **instead** of producing change. Mostly since this is an easy, addictive pastime and producing change requires constant efforts.

There are supposedly know-all psychologists who refer to what appears before the eyes as a shell, which reflects only the outward parts, and the things they believe that are included in the subconsciousness are referred by them as the truth. They know that the concerned mother in facts hates the child and so forth. They will not allow you to confuse them with the facts. I, on the other hand, believe that **the things a person chooses to do in practice testify to his identity choice** and represent him in a more reliable way than a few hidden emotions in his sub-consciousness.

In Friendship School we treat the repression of the present. This repression includes two parameters. The first parameter is **repression of ability**, in the sense of "what can I possibly do? – not in the curious sense but in the desperate sense according to which nothing can be done. This is a person who feels that he cannot do something and tells his friends or his therapist about it. This feeling is perceived as an unchangeable fact, or as a fixed parameter like a person's height. We then accept these facts as a given and we do not even try to change them.

The second parameter is **repression of opportunity**: "there is nowhere to go," "there is nobody to go with" and the like. It is as if someone forcefully covers a person's eyes, and the person cannot see the various possible opportunities.

Removal of repression is done by focusing on the things that can be done, the things that are possible. Even when we refer to the past, we do not do that in order to recall a certain experience, but to recall the <u>ability</u> that was repressed. For instance, someone recalls that once, in the distant past, he rode his bicycles and he finds a friendly usage for this ability in the present; to ride with his children.

We make a distinction between friendly repression and unfriendly repression. A **friendly repression** is an economical act; you forget and repress the things you no longer need – and find time for relating to whatever is relevant at the moment. You must remember that if the brain had not had the ability to repress, we would have been constantly bombarded with countless stimulations which would have prevented us to function. So, it is not such a big deal if you forgot who wrote a certain book, or what an ancient philosopher once said, unless you are a lecturer of literature or philosophy. No one possesses the ability to store unlimited information. Everybody must select the things which are essential to their identity.

In **unfriendly repression** we miss things that are necessary for us - and replace them with irrelevant things . By doing so we damage our abilities and identity. Unfriendly repression is similar to forgetting your own name or address; it is as if you wet your bed. I call this type of repression "a stroke" or "repression of identity." For example, somebody is weeping because of something her mother told her and I say: "I guess you have forgotten the fact that you have boobs and that you are over thirty. If you had not repressed this fact, you would not have felt like a three year old insulted by her mother's predictable words."

Thus, **one should develop means to bypass the automatic components of repression**, in other words, to create bypasses. These bypasses help us to demonstrate a more controlled brain capacity, which includes **exposure** to beneficial opportunities, **screening** and **distinction** between significant and insignificant things. For instance, if it is possible you will forget your spouse's birthday; you should do a friendly deed and write yourself a reminder, so that you will not repress this information. When we do a certain reference activity in our favor time and time again, we find out that it is planted in our consciousness and we do not forget it. For example, if you sing a certain song often, you probably will not forget its words. In Friendship School you will not only deal with your feelings and emotions, and neglect the things you **can** do. For instance, you will not focus on your anxiety and repress the physical closeness of your spouse - on the contrary - you will learn to focus on the caressing, and will very soon sense a pleasure that will drive away the anxiety from your consciousness.

There are numerous approaches that promote the ability to cut off. The ability to internalize and relax. To cut off endless stressful factors.

I recommend **reinforcing the ability to concentrate** and choose. To prefer certain things. **The friendly repression is a companion or the result of our concentration ability**; when the emphasis is put on the thing we choose to focus on, and not on whatever we repress. The mere dealing with a certain domain represses all other domains. The more we sharpen our focusing tools and channel our attention towards the friendly goal, the more we make the best of ourselves. In such a case, we can operate according to our real limitations and not according to the limitations that our impervious brain dictates.

Satisfaction

The feeling we get when our maximal abilities are expressed in the best way.
All of us have quite a few abilities. From time to time we should do an up-do-date bookkeeping and examine the extent to which these abilities are adequately expressed. Many people do not know how to make a distinction between **passing time** and sufficient self-expression. Thus, for instance, we know how to enjoy a movie broadcasted on TV, but if we watch movies all the time we might pass our time pleasantly but we won't get satisfaction since we do not realize our abilities.
If we promote our abilities in an area that enables us to express ourselves enjoyably, we will reach a sufficient solution whose entertaining quality competes with that of the addictive activity which does not cause satisfaction. A social, challenging game such as bridge – or any other enjoyable expression means – easily compete with watching TV.
In Friendship School, passing time serves for recovery between expressive and satisfying actions. After we have used our entire mental budget, we can pass our time reading or watching movies and then it is not considered a waste.

It should be noted that in order to maintain a high level of satisfaction, we should be persistent in relation to scholastic culture. That requires constant development. It is the same characteristic which is found in relation to negative relief. A person who becomes addicted to sleeping pills, needs stronger and stronger pills in order to achieve the desirable outcome. The previous dosage is no longer sufficient. It is also so regarding satisfaction which we define as positive, one must increase his ability more and more. For example, you added another position to your sex life. Good for you. At first it is extremely gratifying. Then it becomes part of the routine and the entertaining quality becomes only reasonable. Thus, one should keep developing friendship even in bed. Whatever you did in the past cannot possibly satisfy you in the future. One must keep learning and developing. This is the real essence of the scholastic culture.

Scenery

All the things that are included in our reservoir of abilities, together with the opportunities spread in front of us. In other words: The things we know how to do and can do and the things that can be achieved in the foreseeable future.

It partially overlaps the term 'spectrum of opportunities'. It means whatever is included in reality before screening. In scholastic culture we recommend that our consciousness scans the scenery. Merely being present without judging or identifying. Without responses of automatic reflexes. Only to scan. We should do that before we respond and identify the things which are relevant for us at a certain moment and choose our direction – like watching the scenery out of a window. A person who looks carefully at the scenery can select a way which will lead him safely towards the most suitable target. Avoiding the scenery means repression which I describe as a kind of blindness or short-sightedness. On the other hand, I compare the brain's control over the repression reflex to improvement of sight, to sharpening of the distinction between various shades. A person who does not notice the multiple opportunities in front of him, is like a person who shuts his eyes and refuses to see the scenery.

A person who does not move, is prepared to see the same scenery over and over. The minimizing of his world makes him very weak: every change in the scenery is bound to destroy his world. He cannot deal with change.

A person who moves, grows, learns or develops – might deal with a changing scenery successfully. His ability changes, his scenery changes accordingly and vice versa: he refers to the changing scenery and his ability changes accordingly. One thing leads to another. The new ability, which is created, enables the exposure to a new scenery, and the exposure to a new scenery expands ability. Learning a new language enables us to produce more in a foreign environment and long exposure to foreign environment contributes to the acquisition of a new language.

When there is movement of growth, a situation that resembles a ride takes place: when we move forward, it seems that the scenery moves backwards. When a woman learns to enjoy living with a spouse and to enjoy children, she will find soon enough that she has left behind all her past friends who remained singles. If they undergo change as well, it is easier to maintain the old friendships.

Students at the Friendship School are asked, among other things, to prepare a list of possibilities and suggestions in order to train their brain to use their specific contextual awareness and understanding: what can serve as a platform for screening and selecting, what is more relevant, what are the priorities.

For instance, someone feels that she detests her husband and is very attracted to a man who is still married but plans to leave his wife. If she is short-sighted, and does not see the scenery, she will act according to this limited data and will probably end up very disappointed. Another woman who sees a more complicated scenery, realizes she has had some stolen moments with a married man which cannot possibly reflect living with him on a daily basis. (Perhaps we should interview his wife in order to find out something about his capabilities as a spouse). Not every single move requires a thorough market survey, but it is advisable to scan the scenery before taking crucial steps.

When our situational understanding is developed, **connections of elements** are created. Let's take for example a woman who meets some guy in the south, with whom she likes to travel; she meets another guy in the north with whom she prefers to have sexual intercourse. She also meets a friend in Jerusalem with whom she likes to talk. This woman spends a lot of energies and produces very little. Another woman would find a guy with whom she likes to have sexual intercourse, travel and talk and then she is left with a mental budget to add to her life other friendly components.

When a person does not repress his various abilities, and in addition sees the scenery, he sees many different scenarios. He can choose the best scenario. This is not a dream, or an imaginary, unrealistic process. It is viewing some scenarios which are all possible and achievable, but at this point of scanning the scenery, we are still not at the production phase. Later on, selecting one of the scenarios, moves the rest of the scenarios to the fringes of the scenery. Such a situation prevents the frustration felt by a person who aims at a certain target in advance, without scanning and obsessively expects and hopes for one thing that might not come true.

Scholastic Culture

A culture which is based primarily on learning and progress.
We produce change through learning. Learning means not to make do with doing things we are used to and love but also to do things

which we have not learnt to love yet. It means doing things you dislike and things that do not suit you. A person who keeps doing only the things he is used to do, tends to re-cycle himself and get stuck in one place. Sometimes he moves sideways instead of forward; namely, he starts building an ability and then neglects it, starts something new – neglects it too and so forth. He tends to abandon the things he has and desire new things. On the other hand, a person who learns something persistently shapes his identity while developing. And if he decides to change his course, he moves from the less to the more, which means that he moves in the direction of something that competes with the thing he already has. For instance, when he changes his workplace, it is not because he does not do a good job, or because he does not like his job, but because he was exposed to a more interesting and rewarding job.

He knows how to use his ability in a certain domain for other domains until he becomes an expert in the new domain as well. He can decide how to combine each of his abilities within his whole identity. He is able to touch a certain subject superficially, and to go deeply into a different subject. He can memorize a musical piece, a book or a poem until these are etched in his mind as if they are inseparable part of his being. He does not need external devices such as a book or a CD player. He can "read" the book from his memory and "hear" the musical piece loudly whenever he wants to. By the way, most people are equipped with this ability. The problem is that they use it to perpetuate negative experiences.

This person knows how to notice other capable people since we can always learn from someone else. He learns to do and to feel what they know and feel. Moreover, he learns his lessons. A person who experiences the same things time and time again, does not learn.

A person of the scholastic culture who has produced a friendly change knows how to maintain it. It is not enough to learn how to drive; you should also get used to driving a car. It is not enough to learn how to play the piano; you must be persistent. It is not enough to lose weight; you should keep in shape. It is not enough to get married; you must refresh your relationship. It is not enough to have children, you should grow with them.

In scholastic culture the person is not locked in a prison of crude judgments unconditionally. If he wants to linger, he does that, from time to time, in order to do a kind of bookkeeping, to examine the important issues and to make sure he does not repress things in an unfriendly manner.

Thus, <u>the ability to learn</u> is the tool that eventually builds the ability to enjoy life and perhaps to get closed to what people call "happiness." People in the scholastic culture learn to express their abilities and talents fully; they know how to learn other people and the cultures of their neighbors. They are equipped with the ability to live. They keep learning till their last day.

Sensational Diagnosis

Diagnosis based on sensations occurs when an individual interprets reality on the basis of his personal sensations.
Many people believe that what they sense and feel reflects the surrounding reality well and expresses their true abilities accurately. Nothing could be further from the truth. Sensational Diagnosis reflects solely the things we were programmed to feel and sense. We learn to sense and feel, and if you wish, even to think, in the same way we learn our mother tongue. We cannot choose where to be born, who our parents are, who our teachers and neighbors will be, nor the stuff they will inject into our brains. Thus, people who are not scholastic will shuffle on and on along the same sensations and emotions rooted in their childhood. They are destined to remain with the same bundle of old experiences and they will reach the same conclusions and judgments time and time again. They will

find it difficult to learn new things, to orientate themselves to the much colorful, complex reality and to interpret it.

Sensational Diagnosis is similar to shortsightedness. The difference is that the short-sighted is aware of the fact that he does not see well. Thus, he will search for means to improve his sight through glasses, microscopes, telescopes etc. The sensational diagnostician will not look for assistance in order to improve the percentages of his sight and comprehension; on the contrary, he will determinedly ward off whatever does not fit his sensations.

The situation gets even more complicated since sometimes what we sense and feel is not necessarily **in**correct. We all know the saying 'Even a broken clock is right twice a day'. Moreover, we sometimes come across an expert who senses the situation accurately even without conducting a thorough examination. For example, an experienced mechanic might identify the failure and know how to fix it just by listening to the engine. Ever since Freud's days feelings and sensations have been the raw material of the common cultural and psychological discourse. We have learnt to report to any kind of audience what we sense and what we feel. "I have the feeling that." "It feels right." "When he told me, I felt that." and so forth.

The therapist will listen with explicit empathy and will be interested in "What else do you feel. Since when have you been feeling this way. What does it do to you. What does it remind you of." This language creates texts such as: "On the one hand I feel that I want to leave him. but on the other hand, I'm scared. And in way I also feel guilty because of the kids."

This type of discourse is based on a built-in belief that if the patient chews his numerous emotions, which are based on the software that was embedded in him during childhood, understands them, digests them and vomits them, reality will change in a certain way. What usually happens is that the patient, instead of achieving change, stays in the same place and is busy recycling his elementary experiences. Of course there is no harm in reviewing the sensational, emotional systems per se. Moreover, some cultures are known to have enforced emotional repression on their subjects, such as the Chinese culture in Mao Tse Tung days, or in the case of a secluded, isolated religious society. In such cultures the subjects become one-dimensional, very repressed or restrained. For these individuals, the mere permission to talk about the secrets of the soul and the open discussion enrich their emotional capabilities and grants them more colorful, complex and mainly human dimensions, and this, in itself, is a friendly deed. <u>Sensational diagnosis may turn into a problematic tool if someone infers the reality from it, and uses it to make cardinal decisions.</u>

" I had a rough time with my husband, I felt I could not take it anymore, and I divorced him. it was tough, but I learned not to be dependent, I learned how to be independent." in most cases with a certain therapeutic support which provided backup for these feelings and even helped the woman in the process of divorce.

She has been on her own for the last decade. She keeps convincing herself that she made the right choice when she decided to get a divorce. But, in fact, she has narrowed down her world. She had more and now she has less (her ex-husband actually remarried and had more children).

Only seldom do we come across an extremely disturbed relationship in which the husband is a violent offender and thus we all agree that the woman is better off without him. But, in most cases, most divorcees were merely involved in a "relationship accident" and were too ignorant to save what they could have had. If they had not judged themselves on the basis of the clashes with their programmed emotional system, but had tried to put these systems aside for a while, and create a different reality, their emotions would have changed "miraculously." I have accompanied couples in conflict numerous times. Instead of discussing their feelings for each other, I sent them to do some homework together and separately. A few weeks later, they became "honeymoon" couples.

Thus, therapies that are based on discussions of what one feels and senses, "what does it do to me" and the like, allow, in most cases, the patient to remain in the same place, to repeat the school year and to recycle himself instead of growing and developing. Or, in the worst-case scenario, support him in making unfriendly decisions.

Is it possible to change, not only the behavior, but also the feelings and emotions?

Yes indeed!

Traditional psychology assumes that a traumatic event must have an impact on our lives, but I see it as learning declination. The problem is not the traumatic event itself, but the habit which was created afterwards and became fixated. Thus we are only dealing with the habit. Moving from abandonment to trust, from anxiety to security – there are, of course lucky individuals that were born into trust and security. All others are supposed to invest in learning and experiencing until their feelings change.

For instance, a motorbike accident. Injury and damage. When the motorist rides his motorbike afterwards he might experience a sense of paralyzing anxiety. Some would let that sense dictate a decision of not riding the motorbike ever again. The response would become fixated and the emotions would dictate avoiding motorbikes altogether. But some people would act completely differently. They would climb the motorbike, increase the speed gradually and soon the sense of anxiety would fade and be replaced by totally different sensations.

(Some would in fact claim that this is an example of learning declination, and not learning one's lessons. Perhaps they are right. This only shows how much the sensational diagnosis and the deriving judgments demand our special attention in order to choose the things which are friendly for us).

In Friendship School the chronic single woman is disqualified from testifying about men. The fact that she came this far without a lifetime partner proves that she does not distinguish the ones who are suitable from those who are unsuitable and she is not able to maintain a relationship. The sensational mechanism that dominates her is misleading and she would find herself attracted to men who have the same limitations and would be disgusted by men who know how to maintain a relationship or be disqualified by them once they realize how limited she is.

A woman who knows how to love, meaning, how to contain another human being, and to maintain a lasting satisfactory relationship with a spouse, a friend, may have a reliable emotional and sensational mechanism. In other words, if she feels repelled by someone, it shows that he is repulsive, in the sense that he has not taken a shower for months and it is really difficult to stand next to him, and not that she has limited love abilities.

In fact, this is the main scope of the learning culture. The ability to acquire an ability which was not part of your culture, or your "early programming," and the ability to create an emotional, sensational change. For instance, riding a motorbike. (I always recommend taking lessons in riding motorbikes. Probably because I am an addict myself, but mainly because it enables one to produce **rapid change learning**, sometime during the course of a single lesson. She (apparently, for some reason, I recommend it more to women than to men. Especially to women who did not ride bicycles or rollerblades) climbs on the motorbike in the first lesson, terrified, and within minutes her fear turns into an almost childlike pleasure. More than once the ones who experienced this emotional, sensational change understand from this simple experience that it is possible to create change through an intentional act and this understanding is reflected in other areas in which changes are needed). Similarly, disgust turns into affection and amongst scholastics feelings of hatred turn into love.

We will expand a little on "how" learning is accomplished and how it is done. **Sensational diagnosis decreases the chance of learning new and different things.** For example, a person who was trained to be disgusted by seafood sits in front of a plate of shrimp in garlic-butter dressing. Epicures know that it is absolutely delicious, but our hero would probably feel nothing but disgust. This sensation is totally predictable considering the way he was raised. If he concludes, according to his senses that "it," the dish, is disgusting, it means that his sensational mechanism stupefies his brain. In this case, the damage is not great and he would remain accustomed to the eating habits he learned from his mother. Similarly, the chronic single woman feels disgusted or bored by the man who tries to win her affection, disqualifies him and remains single.

However, the scholastic recognizes his feelings of disgust as well, but assumes they derive from the way he was brought up and does not diagnose the food according to these sensations. He assumes that the dish is tasty since he looks around and sees other people who eat it delightedly. Thus, an individual who wishes to have better chances of making a change, must bypass his emotions and try to learn how to enjoy shrimp in garlic butter dressing. In other words, to concentrate on the taste of the dish. It is obvious that if he keeps concentrating on the predictable sensations, he prevents himself from knowing anything about the food on his plate. Only when he manages to put aside his predictable sensations as a disturbing factor does his improved concentration enable him to sense some of the taste. There is no doubt that the old, familiar sensations, like a mother tongue, still live at the back of his mind. But he would concentrate on the remote sensation of the food's taste. He would notice that the taste had changed a little. Surely, the dish is still not tasty, but does not cause utter disgust. From now on he should concentrate on the little changes in the sensations derived from the dish. Meaning that from time to time it becomes easier for him to eat it, and later on, easier, until at last he finds it really delicious. Change accomplished. The sense of disgust turned into pleasure. He understands that the attempt of producing a change cannot possibly be unique. Each type of learning requires a certain amount of time and effort. Now he is free to make more and more desirable changes in his life.

Anyone can, with a certain amount of effort, recall and recognize in his reservoir a change in the sensation towards something in the course of his life. In most cases it happened since a person was caught in certain circumstances that brought about the change. In Friendship School, however, instead of leaving it for chance or pure luck, we will **initiate** the change.

In Friendship School I will not ask what you feel, but what have you done so far. If I interest myself in deeds, I will learn a lot about feelings. Feelings are the outcome of ability. Ability is the outcome of experiencing. I will be interested in sensational shift and change of feelings in the course of the learning experiences.

I call the above production of change a <u>bypass</u> of sensational diagnosis.

Another tool for producing mental and sensational change is the ability to cognitively recognize various situations and gain greater understanding from them. This ability aids in improving the ability of scanning a wider array of sensations and feelings which leads to a more solid reasoning. For example, at this moment you are really furious with your husband, your whole being screams to kick him out of your life permanently. If you move your consciousness backwards and forwards, you will remember the positive, exciting experiences you have had with this man, and notice what the future may hold for both of you and remain a friend of this person whose presence is irritating you at this moment. And vice versa. You live with a disturbed person who is a criminal and violent against you. You know that you must run for your life, but at this moment he is calling you sweetheart, giving you a piece of jewelry and you mellow down. But if you scan the wider array and understand that he has not really changed, you will not change your decision.

Another tool is what I call the <u>language of facts</u>. I use my ability to view and understand a specific context and mediate between my client and his world. (For instance, she reports **a sense** of great disappointment at her spouse and her disappointment provides evidence that he is an awful man. Sometimes, it is not true. I know him personally. In such a case I might say to her: "He is not disappointing. It is you who do not notice him. You expect precisely what he is unable to give, and you miss what he is able and wants to give you. It is as if you enter a bookstore when you actually need vegetables. You would probably go out emptyhanded. Not because the store is disappointing, but because you did not pay attention to the goods in the store. Feelings of insult which appear frequently are, in most cases, a result of a sort of sight defect. When one improves his sight, he learns how to produce change in the other person, or how not to expect what cannot be changed.

Our learning efforts are endless. We must sharpen our learning tools consistently, catch up, learn our lessons, improve what needs to be improved; we must learn to ask ourselves what we should add to our lives – in order to achieve a reliable tool for world orientation. In short, in 'Friendship School' we will not focus on what one feels like doing but on what one **should** do.

State of Aggregation

The up-to-date information regarding our abilities at a given time.
This is a reliable reflection of the reservoir of abilities each one of

us has. It enables us to know the exact level of each one of us in various areas.

In order to learn about a person we should ask him what he is doing and what he used to do in the past. A detailed answer to these questions will provide us with more reliable information than assessments and judgments. If we add to it knowledge about his days' content, namely, what he does with his time – we will be able to know what the level of his current ability is in every domain according to the amount of time he dedicates to each of his occupations.

You might want to think of the identity as a cake which is divided into several pieces, some of which are large, some of which are small, and some of which are really thin.

Examine the size of the professional piece and the size of the rest of the pieces: relationship, family, hobbies, etc. Pay attention to the connections between the pieces. Do they live peacefully side by side or are they at odds with each other? Examine the cake as a whole. Is it fixated or is it constantly moving? New abilities are added from time to time; one ability fades away and each movement changes the whole identity.

If you learn how to do it you will be able to know who the person who stands in front of you is. Your knowledge will not be perfect, you will never be able to know another person completely, but you will have a reliable tool of knowing people which is better than many other diagnostic tools.

A state of aggregation is not a crude psychological diagnosis; it is not a diagnosis at all, but it can serve as the basis for a discussion about the things which are worthy of promotion and the things which are not, and how to move forward. This is the foundation of building a personal learning program.

On top of this foundation we build a plan of various types of friendly homework, for each person according to his best interest. Addition of abilities eventually creates change and shapes identities.

Symptom

A phenomenon that reflects the disturbing of balance in our inner world.

When we are exposed to things which already exist in our reservoir of abilities, there are no symptoms; but when we are faced with a new element, our organism reacts in different ways. In a non-scholastic culture, the symptoms are fixated and sometimes become the center of identity, so that some people define themselves on the basis of their symptoms: "I am asthmatic"; "I am dyslectic"; "I am disabled"; "I am sick."

Canonical psychology, being a part of the trampled culture, ascribes considerable, almost exclusive, weight to symptoms. According to the traditional order, we must mark the problem, understand its origins, remove it and only then we are ready to move on. But the truth is that these traditional stages require enormous effort which causes damage to the patients' identity – the patients shape their identity as people who have problems and need to be treated.

On the other hand, scholastic culture does not focus on the symptoms at all. Instead of "I am disabled" – a crude, somewhat negative definition, we would say "I am a one-legged person," which is a factual saying, namely, noting a fact rather than defining identity. However, it is not sufficient. It is very important where you place this information within your identity. When you say "I," and add your main occupation, such as electrical engineer, married with children, and somewhere at the end of the list you mention that you have only one leg, you refer to your identity in a friendly manner. However, when your list starts with "I am a one-legged person," or when there is not even a list following this definition, it is as if you say that you have nothing else to offer. That is who I am, like a beggar who emphasizes his deformity in order to get more donations. An accurate reference to the missing leg is one that prevents a person from shaping his identity as a professional football player, but allows him to shape numerous other identities.

Thus, the scholastic culture does not dwell on "treating" the symptoms, but deals with **production** of change and acquisition of new abilities. These abilities might even **compensate** for the disability. Shaping such a person's identity, like shaping any other person's identity, is based on the abilities in various states of aggregations and not on the disabilities. As mentioned above, the first stage of learning how to acquire a new ability is sometimes difficult and a few symptoms might appear: but later on, when the new ability is internalized and takes its place alongside other abilities, the symptoms disappear. Thus, the symptoms are expected side effects that might accompany the first stage of change or learning, but only at the beginning. They resemble calluses on the hands of a person who is not used to hard work, or the anxiety of a person who is about to go on stage for the first time in his life. If we do not dwell or focus on the symptoms, but keep learning and experiencing patiently and gradually, the ability improves and the symptoms disappear and give way to pleasure which is deerived from expressing our abilities.

See: "Dealing with problems," "Crude Rejection" and "Bypass."

In a non-scholastic culture the symptom might turn into crude rejection means of all other possibilities. A person crudely claims that he is disabled, perceives that as a fact and no longer attempts to make a change.

Technology

An optimistic concept which means a change following performance.

The ability to produce change originates in several sources. The best source is being lucky and born into a culture that develops abilities and nurtures freedom of choice. Other possible sources are adapting friendly thinking and using it in order to make a change in a certain area. But, there is another way that does not include friendly thinking: **to precede thinking and feeling with doing**. That is what I call technology.

Throughout the years, I have seen many people who have made enormous changes even without a broad scenery sight and developing friendly thinking. These people were willing to learn and simply agreed to do their <u>homework</u> in the spirit of the famous saying in Judaism: "We will do and we will listen" but in the midst of doing, they find, to their surprise, that their mental system has undergone change. That means that many things they learnt in "Friendship School" were internalized and became important components of their identity. Technology bore fruit and understating came, if at all, at a later stage. It often happens in reality without an overt prior intention. For example, a young husband who feels he is not mature enough to be a father, but somehow becomes a parent. And so, after a while he becomes an enthusiastic father who is attached to his baby boy and loves him profoundly.

Unfortunately, it does not necessarily develop this way. Some people agree to experience for a while but eventually rejects the opportunity for change. Their original programming wins and they remain as disabled as they used to be. They keep on saying: "OK, I'll keep dating her but I don't feel I love her." Thus, the agreement to function and perform certain activities in a behavioristic manner does not always lead to a complete, profound change. The organ responsible for changes and feelings is, after all, the brain. If the person does not concentrate well enough on the relevant stimulus, he will not be able to produce pleasure and excitement.

Try to scan the activities that bring you joy. You will find out that many of them crept in your life not because you wanted to deal with them, but because you were dragged into them. Somehow you learn how to like these activities which become part of your identity, namely, yours. In "Friendship School" we prefer to initiate the worthy elements and not to leave it to mere chance.

Many **singles** who started dating arbitrarily as part of their homework became loving spouses. It is hard to define when a person moves from a technical performance to real joy. People differ in this sense. When a person tramples in his inability, he perpetuates the existing situation. But when a person discovers the ability to make a profound, emotional change, it usually leads to a chain of additional changes. When the first change takes place the person himself is surprised by the change in his feelings and emotions. Then he starts looking for other places where change is needed and makes additional changes. Now he is already equipped with a reliable tool. He knows that whenever he decides to add an ability, he will make the effort and the result will probably be positive. He has joined the scholastic culture. Thus, technology, sometimes, is highly productive.

See: "Production," "Homework," "Day's Contents."

Trampled Culture (Culture of Diagnosis & Judgment)

The manner of observing which accompanies almost any human reference. The way we keep examining things according to the criteria we have known all our lives.

The phenomenon of trampling is so common that most people cannot make a distinction between a fact and a judgment. When they repeat the same judgment over and over again, they perceive it as a solid fact. From then on, there is not much of a chance of additional information sinking in and changing the things they already "know." I see it as "brain damage." It derives from the way we were educated by our parents, and teachers who stuffed judgments into our brain, instead of giving us thinking tools that would prepare our brain to contain colorful, diversified scenery and not to lock every piece of information in a slot of preconception. It is difficult to describe the extent of the brain damage caused by the judgmental culture. Many doctors do not see the person in front of them; they see a case characterized by a certain disease. Many mistakes are made because of that approach. Obviously, diagnosis is an important phase of healing, but it should be done only after an observation of the patient himself, and not only through the written words.

Psychology, which attempted to become science, has copied this approach from medicine, and burdened itself with endless diagnosis. There are monstrous books which deal with infinite collections of symptoms and diagnosis. A catalogue of metal types or sorting out potatoes might help us sometime to organize things; and organization can be a friendly thing. But an attempt to categorize people is similar to locking them in a thinking dungeon, or trying to get an elephant into a Mini. Moreover, the diagnosis and the dealing with the problems usually become a cause of fixation and of frustrating trampling – dwelling on the past, the emotions, the dreams – which ultimately does not lead us anywhere. Only if we become members of the scholastic culture, and refer mainly to the present and the future, and less to the past, will we be able to change.

Other products of the trampled culture are, amongst other things, religion (any religion), blind admiration of a leader or a superstar, and the thing I refer to as "automatic programming" – performing activities which require thought without such thought; for instance, people who vote for a certain political party only because they are used to voting for it.

Working Meetings

Meetings of the guide and the client for the purpose of accompanying the process of change.

These meetings take place after we define the language we speak, the schedule and the abilities to be promoted. The meetings are very practical and their purpose is to achieve well-defined goals. During the meetings we go over the homework with the client and decide what his homework for the next meeting will be. The number of the meetings depends on the individual client. The pace of progress is also totally personal. However, usually only several meetings are needed.